D0907070

ALCOHOL IN *HUMAN VIOLENCE*

THE GUILFORD SUBSTANCE ABUSE SERIES

Editors

HOWARD T. BLANE, Ph.D.

Research Institute on Alcoholism, Buffalo

THOMAS R. KOSTEN, M.D.

Yale University School of Medicine, New Haven

ALCOHOL IN HUMAN VIOLENCE

Kai Pernanen
University of Uppsala, Sweden

Foreword by
Dwight B. Heath
Brown University

THE GUILFORD PRESS
New York London

A Division of Guilford Publications, Inc.
72 Spring Street, New York, NY 10012

Printed in the United States of America

This book is printed on acid-free paper.

Last digit is print number: 9 8 7 6 5 4 3 2 1

Library of Congress Cataloging-in-Publication Data

Pernanen, Kai.
Alcohol in human violence / Kai Pernanen.
p. cm. — (The Guilford substance abuse series)
Includes bibliographical references and index.
ISBN 0-89862-171-2
1. Alcoholism and crime. 2. Violence. 3. Alcoholism—Psychological aspects. I. Title. II. Series.
[DNLM: 1. Alcohol Drinking. 2. Violence. WM 274 P452a]
HV5053.P45 1991
364.2′4—dc20
DNLM/DLC
for Library of Congress 91-16338
CIP

Foreword

In this last decade of the 20th century, alcohol is very much a focus of both research and the mass media throughout much of the world. The same is true of human violence. Unfortunately, many researchers and journalists presume that alcohol and violence are inextricably linked and this presumption has become a truism in the minds of many. Kai Pernanen's book is important, both empirically and theoretically, as a counter to such glib—and inaccurate—generalization. It should help readers understand some of the complexity and subtlety of the interaction between ethanol and the human organism—a systematic interaction in which psychological and social variables are as important as biochemical and neuropharmacological ones. It should also help readers understand the complexity of motivations and antecedents to violence, among which alcohol is not only unspecific but also relatively rare in comparison with many other variables.

As an anthropologist, I consider it important to point out that the association that is often posited between alcohol and violence should be viewed as a "missing" link: a link that superficially appears logical and is easily reinforced by conventional ways of thinking and speaking, but that nevertheless remains to be explained and, for that matter, has not yet been fully proven by the systematic compilation and evaluation of empirical data.

More generally, there is an ease with which we accept the appropriateness of linkages between words within their social contexts, whether they denote the concrete and banal or the symbolic and sublime. "Gin and tonic" somehow seem in place on the veranda, and "coffee and donuts" are the traditional fare during breaks at conferences. "Damon and Pythias" have long epitomized companionship, and "love and marriage"—as celebrated in a popular song that ironically became outdated in just a few years—"go together like a horse and carriage." These examples of linkages are not frivolous, but exemplify an important anthropological insight: There is nothing intrinsic or natural about any of these linkages; they are all cultural conventions, meaningful in limited contexts because members of specific social groups tend to have common understandings about many things in the world around them.

Such shared understandings often come to be called "folk wisdom" or "common sense" and are mistakenly thought to have "objective reality," or to reflect a universal "human nature." But even with those homely examples of such links, cultural change has prompted us to reconsider what used to be a compelling logic of association. In recent decades, "coffee and donuts" have been replaced in many contexts by more healthful or fashionable refreshments; similarly "gin and tonic" has given way to "wine and cheese," "burger and shake," or "beer and pizza," in their own socially defined environments. A younger generation, although ostensibly more accepting of gay rights and homosexual partnerships, may never have heard of Damon and Pythias. Furthermore, "love and marriage" have proven to be just as separable, if not quite as scarce, as a horse and carriage. All of these shifts have occurred within the memory of individuals, some of whom appear to have sincerely believed the lyrics of that song when it was popular in the 1950s. In this roundabout—but effective, I hope—demonstration it is evident that the logic of many seemingly "natural" linkages is not at all intrinsic or inherent, but rather is a cultural artifact. As such, the logic of conventional linkages can change within a given culture over time, as we have seen; it is also likely to differ from culture to culture at any given time.

One of the special strengths of Pernanen's work is that it includes a transnational (some would say cross-cultural) perspective on the subject. The richest data derive from his intensive study of a Canadian community, a sort of "natural experiment" for the analysis of both alcohol use and human aggression. But these data are set within a broader context by frequent comparisons and contrasts with related information from Scandinavia and from the United States, where most of the studies on social correlates of drinking have been conducted.

Another unusual and significant feature of this book is what might be called "triangulation." Rather than starting from the premise that alcohol and violence are "naturally" linked and studying police records, hospitalizations, or other sources that were compiled with very different purposes in mind, he went to the general population in a natural community and built on their workaday experiences with alcohol and, quite distinctively, also with violence. The importance of his having "broken the link" is evident in the striking finding that, for most of the people he surveyed, "other types of affective behavior typically predominate in alcohol use situations." In fact, the most common was "behavior usually linked to positive affect" (p. 199). Such occurrences are obviously not so well documented by the media or by public agencies as are violent encounters, but the weight of human experience must not be ignored.

Furthermore, he notes, "Some alcohol-induced processes actually decrease the likelihood of physical aggression . . ." (p. 222). By fixing our attention on a particular kind of outcome, drinking is often thought to "trigger" violence in an almost automatic way, although the opposite reaction actually appears to be more often the case. Much of our perception depends upon what Pernanen calls the "moral framing" of what happens.

It is in terms of framing that he makes another unusual contribution, by showing how the same acts that would be viewed with alarm if someone were hurt are often reported in the media as humorous when there is no damage done.

The rich corpus of data on what happens when, in the normal course of events, people drink, and the related but separable data on what, in the normal course of events, leads to violence, offer many new insights into human behavior. The author's refusal to fit those data into theoretical and conceptual formulations that he finds inadequate and his imaginative integration of a cognitive perspective make this a refreshingly innovative account that should have considerable impact on thinking about the subjects for years to come.

DWIGHT B. HEATH
Brown University

Acknowledgments

The empirical research project reported in this book was funded by the Promotion and Prevention Directorate of Health and Welfare Canada (RODA Grant 1212-5-236). The active support of Dr. Irving Rootman is remembered with gratitude. The Addiction Research Foundation of Ontario administered the funds and provided other much appreciated day-to-day resources including office space and secretarial assistance. Dr. Wolfgang Schmidt was instrumental in bringing about this support. The Thunder Bay Regional Office of the same foundation assisted during the lengthy field work stage of the project.

The forty-one interviewers who carried out the fieldwork for the interview survey, in at times difficult conditions during a northern Ontario winter, naturally deserve a great deal of credit for the theoretical and practical impact that this study may have.

The systematic observations that were carried out in 28 taverns and bars of the study community are dealt with in this book only for the purpose of extracting naturalistic insights and providing real-life illustrations to the findings. However, since the aims of the total study in the community formed an integrated whole and several of the ideas expressed in this book have their roots in what was learned in the observations of drinking behavior, the contribution of the 12 observers who helped us gather data is also central to the present work.

Police Chiefs Onni Harty and Tom R. Keep and Planning and Research Officer Gary Lowry of the Thunder Bay Police Force made possible the use of police records of violent crime that occurred in the community. This helped the study gain additional depth.

The capable assistance of Kerstin Carsjö has been of vital importance throughout every phase of the project. Ron Kerr, who helped with the coding and processing of data provided a steadying influence on the project. Tuija Puiras and Marc Metsāranta helped us commendably in supervising the interviews and observations. Toivo Pōysä of the Finnish

Social Research Institute of Alcohol Studies shared with us his unique expertise in the field of social survey research.

In translating our sometimes vague analytical requests into a precise and still flexible format for computer processing we could not have wished for better expertise than that of Henzel Jupiter of the Addiction Research Foundation. Several members of the staff of the Department of Social Medicine at the University of Uppsala have assisted in later analyses of the Canadian data.

In any major undertaking a combination of practical help and generous moral support are vital ingredients. Paulette Walters, who typed and edited the scientific reports that form the basis of this book, gave us both of these at a time when they were truly needed.

In a freelancing researcher's life there are typically recurrent periods of hiatus in funding. These must be filled with work that is not directly related to his main interests, and assistance for research work is hard to come by. If he is lucky, members of his family will step in during such periods and do some of the work normally done by secretaries or research assistants. I am grateful to my daughter Satu for help in several stages of the project.

Within the social study of human behavior there are no better ways of approaching central objectives, be they descriptive, assessment oriented, or explanatory, than by replicating studies systematically in contexts that differ culturally and/or structurally. I am fortunate in that the study reported here is being replicated in a Swedish community, at the time of this writing. For this work and some remaining statistical analyses of the Canadian data I have received financial support from the Swedish Commission for Social Research (Grants D84/211 and D87/82) and the Swedish Alcohol Research Fund (Grant 87/27). Some of the theoretical ideas presented in the book also evolved under their auspices. The Swedish Council for Planning and Coordination of Research has provided financial means for theoretical work in the area of alcohol use and violence (Grant 880383: 3/A 9-4-5). This has provided the peace of mind acutely needed if such work is to succeed. Although most of the fruits of this labor will be reported in a subsequent monograph, some central theoretical and metatheoretical ideas from this effort are included in the present book.

The active and moral support of Orvar Olsson, Claes-Göran Westrin and Vera Novakova during the Swedish study should also be mentioned. They have meant much in helping the author continue this line of research.

Two research colleagues have provided penetrating and useful comments on a next-to-final manuscript: Colin G. Miles, chief psychologist with the Kingston Penitentiary Treatment Unit in Ontario, Canada, and

Jussi Simpura, director of the Social Research Institute of Alcohol Studies in Helsinki, Finland. They of course bear no responsibility for remaining flaws.

Finally, I want to thank Anna Brackett and Marie Sprayberry for the thorough and sensitive editing of my manuscript and for escorting it through the publishing process.

Contents

ALCOHOL IN HUMAN VIOLENCE

1

Introduction and Pre-Empirical Considerations

CONCEPTUAL BACKGROUND AND PURPOSES OF THE PRESENT RESEARCH

The study reported in this book was undertaken in order to provide both more empirical depth and wider theoretical scope to questions regarding the relationships between drinking and aggression. Hitherto, almost the only means of investigating naturally occurring connections between alcohol use and aggression in a systematic and quantified way has been the analysis of official records of violent crime. There are both practical and conceptual problems with the use of such official documentation for theoretical and descriptive purposes, and some of these are discussed in this book. Specifically, because of the potential biases and information gaps inherent in these sources, general population studies with more depth and detail in the data collected are badly needed. Attempts at integration of empirical approaches also need to be made. These approaches should include social survey-based studies, experimental research, and observational studies in natural settings, to mention a few of the more obvious ones. In theoretical developments, too, we need an integration of approaches. The field is unnecessarily scattered.

Another consideration that led to the present study is the conviction that situational factors relevant in establishing statistical links between alcohol use and aggressive behavior can be studied using social-scientific methodology. At the same time, I feel that firmer empirical and theoretical connections to experimental psychology can be established through this type of study. For this purpose, episodes of relatively mild forms of natural aggression have been included, and their relationship to drinking has been established by means traditional to sociological inquiry.

Central conceptual themes that are necessary for an understanding of the processes linking alcohol and aggressive behavior are discussed fairly extensively. They are important for appreciating the cognitive frameworks that limit the perceptions of the scientist, the casual observer, and the average person alike. They in part determine general boundaries of the present state of knowledge in the field of violence, in the study of alcohol use, and in their intersection, which is the topic of this book. One of these cognitive frameworks is discussed in this introductory chapter. Another cluster of conceptual issues is discussed in the final chapter, where the broad outline of a multidisciplinary theory of alcohol-related aggression is presented. The conceptual themes discussed can be called "pre-empirical"; in the main, they are linguistic and cognitive, and not specific to the problem of alcohol's connections with aggressive behavior. Because of the dual nature of intoxicated behavior as both human goal-directed conduct and pharmacological determination, however, they come out comparatively clearly in the present context.[1]

Perhaps the best way to become aware of the cognitive boundary conditions that currently define the subject matter in the study of alcohol-related violence, and above all that shape the theoretical explanations in this area, would be close naturalistic observations of (1) behavior "under the influence of" alcohol and (2) episodes of human aggression. Naturalistic contemplation—as free as humanly possible of paradigmatic assumptions and prejudices—is especially crucial when one deals with largely unexplored phenomena, such as the connections between alcohol use and aggression. In part, the need for greater naturalistic impact in the general study of human motivation and behavior has been expressed as a need for "taking the problem of description seriously" (Forgas, 1979, p. 29), as part of the effort to provide unbiased material for the later creative effort of hypothesis formation and theory construction. Only after the descriptive stage should we enter into critical testing of hypotheses. This is now an agreed-upon agenda, at

1. Still other conceptual and cognitive themes will be discussed in a planned monograph focusing on the inception of anger and conflict, and on the role of alcohol in these processes. This monograph will also present a more detailed theory of alcohol's links with the escalation of anger and conflict into aggression and physical violence. It will be argued that in order for such a theory to be valid, it must rest on a general theory of the effects of alcohol on cognition and behavior.

least in programmatic treatises of social psychology (Forgas, 1979; McGuire, 1973; Warr, 1977). In the study of the relationship between alcohol use and aggressive behavior, we have not yet reached the stage of growing agreement on the importance of description in order to study essential social aspects of intoxicated behavior. The predominant approach is still, to use the words of Warr (1977) when discussing general social psychology, "predominantly mechanistic, individualistic and pure," and it "gives excessive weight to only a small part of our subject matter" (p. 2).

In this introductory chapter and in the concluding theoretical discussion in Chapter 9, I try perhaps the next best thing to naive naturalism making use of direct observation of drunken behavior: I attempt to bring forth hidden conceptual issues and prevailing cognitive frames by discussing written illustrations of alcohol-related behavior from the mass media. The ways in which the individual journalists and editors, and we as readers, react to and cognitively handle the information contained in these illustrations is illuminating.

Description is thus an important goal in itself. It is approached in the research described in this book through an investigation of naturally occurring episodes of aggression, and, to a much lesser extent, a supplementary examination of drinking situations. However, both description and theory construction must also be put into a general cognitive (in part, epistemological) framework, and I attempt to do this as well. Explanations of drunken comportment are not independent of common tacit assumptions regarding human nature and human behavior. As researchers, we should be aware of our own human cognitive limitations and of the cognitive frames that determine our categorizations and attempts at explanations of phenomena. In part, the same categorizations and types of explanations guide the acting and interacting individuals whose behavior we are trying to explain (Winch, 1958).

Unfortunately, prejudicial "scientific" paradigms often prematurely structure the research questions asked, and thereby curb (and to some extent confuse) research and theory pertaining to the linkage between alcohol use and aggression. The field has been in the grip of a framework derived from the natural sciences, with little alternative input from more "humanistic" paradigms. I briefly argue the thesis that there need be no contradiction between the two, and that they meet unproblematically in concrete empirical sequences of action and interaction.

Somewhat unexpectedly, what has become most clearly evident during the course of the fieldwork and the analysis of data (in part reported here) is the importance of social definitions and interactional processes in mediating, through confluent cognitive and cultural processes, both alcohol use and aggression. This type of serendipity that forces the importance of sociocultural factors upon us is not unique in the study of alcohol-related behavior (see Heath, 1988c). The strong grip of natural-scientific explanatory paradigms no doubt underlies such feelings of mild surprise.

These largely programmatic ideas on greater methodological, empirical, and theoretical integration in studying alcohol-related aggression have to be kept in mind for the foreseeable future as heuristic orientations. For the time being, we still need a much firmer empirical foothold, in order to assess the validity of the relationship between alcohol use and violence in potentially less biased samples of violence episodes and of actors in these episodes than those available in official documents. We need information on the potential role of alcohol in the choice of different types of violent acts and in escalations in the seriousness of aggression and physical violence, as well as in the use of indiscriminate aggression in partial or total obliviousness to the nature of the victim, the setting, and the general social context. We also need very basic data on variations in aggregate strengths of the overall relationship between alcohol use and aggression in different population groups and in different types of drinking situations, as well as information regarding what types of interactional processes and resolutions of milder aggressive flareups are more likely when one person has been drinking as compared to when neither has been drinking or when both have been drinking. These are all only a few items that a more detailed research agenda might include. In the main, this book is an attempt to achieve some of these mainly descriptive objectives (in a still somewhat piecemeal fashion) by means of empirical data from an intensive study of the connections between alcohol use and aggressive behavior. The study was carried out in a Canadian community between the years 1977 and 1981.

MORAL AND COGNITIVE FRAMEWORKS FOR INTOXICATED BEHAVIOR

Before discussing two basic cognitive frameworks for the conceptualization of human behavior in general and intoxicated behavior in particular, I briefly consider the *moral* framework for a couple of alcohol-related problem areas. Moral framings typically in part derive from the assessment of several different cognitive frameworks, which makes their analysis more intricate. Moral assessments may *seem* simpler because of the great practice we all have with moral issues from our everyday contexts, and our tendency to simplify morality through cognitive stereotyping.

Several researchers speak of the cultural ambivalence toward alcohol that is found in many societies (Ahlström-Laakso, 1973; Meyerson,

1959; Pittman, 1967; Room, 1976), particularly the Protestant parts of the Western world. This ambivalence is partly reflected in, and sustained by, prevailing views on the serious phenomena linked to alcohol use.

Drunken driving and its consequences form one of the major clusters in the determination of attitudes toward alcohol use. It has always been in the public eye, partly, no doubt, because the population at risk of becoming an offender is so large—in fact, almost coextensive with the large segment of the population who are not teetotalers and who also drive cars. The population at risk of becoming *victims* of impaired driving is even larger and even more unselected. This risk is felt to be largely independent of any selective criteria of morality or responsibility. No factors that would lessen the perceived loss and injustice to the victims and their intimates can be applied, since a significant proportion of the moral blame or technical faults cannot be assigned to the victims. This nonselective nature of risk makes it easy to identify with those involved in drinking and driving, both as potential victims and to some extent as potential culprits. Organized forms of public outrage—for example, parents' groups such as Mothers Against Drunk Driving (MADD), mainly aimed at the traditionally light sentences meted out to drunken drivers in North America—derive considerable social salience and organizational power from having such an amorphous potential constituency of victims and their intimates.

Except for drunken driving, the public concerns and moral assessments related to alcohol use in North America have traditionally been related to the nonsituational aspects of use, and above all to alcoholism—its moral and medical status, and its prevention and treatment. Concern about longer-term consequences has lately also focused specifically on the fetal alcohol syndrome, and more generally on the much wider problem area of what alcohol use in a society means to its public health.

However, in all the public defining process of the causal role and moral status of alcohol in North American society, and in the parallel molding of public attitudes toward the substance, comparatively little reference has been made to the role of alcohol in violence. Similarly, astonishingly little has been said about this role in the public debate on violent crime and discussions on family violence. The general public and the helping professions alike have been disposed to viewing violence in the family as a private matter (e.g., Straus, 1986a). In the studies of domestic violence that have come about despite such widespread attitudes, alcohol still seems very much a minor issue (see the review by Epstein, Cameron, & Room, 1977), although this lack of emphasis has been changing over the last decade and a half (e.g., see Amaro, Fried, Cabral, & Zuckerman, 1990; Behling, 1979; Byles, 1978, 1980; Carlson,

1977; Eberle, 1982; Gerson, 1978; Hindman, 1977; Miller, Downs, & Gondoli, 1989; Richardson, 1980; Roy, 1977; Van Hasselt, Morrison, & Bellack, 1985). If we consider the extent to which alcohol is statistically implicated in violent crime, the traditional paucity of interest in the role of alcohol in North American violence is surprising. In the discussion to follow on the cognitive structures applied to drunken behavior, we may find a partial explanation for this fact in the cognitively ambiguous and emotionally ambivalent way in which alcohol use and socially visible drunken behavior are perceived.

Another part of the explanation for the lack of public outrage with regard to violent behavior under the influence of alcohol probably resides in the fact that the victims of violence in alcohol use contexts seem more closely selected on morally relevant criteria than are, for example, victims of drunken driving. High-risk situations for violence are generally perceived as containing mostly people who know full well about the context and its inherent risks. They often drink themselves. In this way, the social-interactional context taints victims as well as assailants. A common stereotypical representation of alcohol-related aggression is a free-for-all, a "drunken brawl," in a place where excessive drinking is condoned and where it is exceedingly hard at times to make a distinction between a culprit and a victim. This makes identification with the victim comparatively difficult.

There are great variations even among Western nations in the extent to which beliefs related to alcohol's role in aggression have shaped views of the moral status of alcohol. In the Scandinavian countries (especially Finland, Norway, and Sweden), unlike North America, violence has been one of the main concerns in shaping attitudes toward alcohol use. The two phenomena have been seen as almost inextricably linked, to the extent that general statistical data on violent crime have been used as indicators of the total "alcohol situation" in Finland. In other European countries, especially those in southern Europe, such perceptions are not at all central. The differences in emphasis are no doubt due to differences in the prevalence of alcohol-related aggression in different countries. They are to some extent reflected in the volume of research carried out in the area of alcohol use and aggression.

The lack of public concern about drinking and aggression in North America may also result to some extent from the fact that the moral framework for aggression (like that for alcohol use) varies greatly, depending on the context. (Pronounced dependence on context may in fact be the essence of ambivalence in attitudes.) On the one hand, an aggressive stance is considered desirable in many general undertakings and specific situations, such as in business, politics, and sports. On the other hand, it is circumscribed by intricate formal and informal social rules and expectations, and is totally condemned in many social contexts.

Finally, there is a more general type of ambivalent vacillation involved in the perception and explanation of (as well as in reactions to) drunken aggression. This is related to the way in which we view the determination of a drinking person's behavior. It coincides with a central conceptual tension in the scientific explanation of human behavior generally. It is very prominent in our way of viewing and explaining behavior under the influence of alcohol; here, it has some interesting consequences. I illustrate this tension in the next section by studying the mass media's reactions (and our probable reactions as readers) to various types of behavior after drinking. These reactions provide some data for a quasi-naturalistic study of pre-empirical factors that guide explanations of human behavior in connection with alcohol use. Such factors underlie an unnecessary bifurcation in the explanation of drinking-related aggression. Human categorizations of reality and the selection of explanatory metaparadigms are central concerns in this discussion.

EXPLANATIONS FOR DRINKING-RELATED BEHAVIOR: GOAL-DIRECTEDNESS VERSUS DETERMINATION BY NATURAL FORCES

Tension between the Two Frameworks: Evidence from News Reports

If drunken aggression does not have very serious consequences, it is often seen in a humorous mode, as part of "the crazy things that drunks do." This interpretive framework is especially likely to come into play if more than one intoxicated person is involved—when, for instance, group interaction evolves into a "drunken brawl." Staged versions from television and the movies no doubt help shape our conceptions about drunken violence. Relatively few of us have seen a saloon fight, but if asked to describe one we would probably know the exact ingredients. At times, however, fact seems to equal fiction:

> COBOURG [, Ontario] (CP)—Five members of a railway work gang and a local man were in court yesterday on charges ranging from assault to escaping custody after a chair-tossing brawl in a bar spilled into the streets during the weekend.
>
> Seventeen police officers drawn from area forces needed two hours early Sunday to bring the roisterers—who marched on the stationhouse at one point—under control.

> Police said yesterday that the opening round of the incident occurred Friday night when 25 members of a railway work gang paid a visit to a hotel beverage parlor. Three men were evicted after a disturbance and the crew returned Saturday with revenge in mind, police said.
>
> Chairs, tables and glassware were flying when Cobourg police stepped in. Two blocks were cordoned off as the donnybrook churned into the street.
>
> The brawlers attempted to re-enter the bar but it was locked, so five men marched on the police station and got as far as the outer office before the dispatcher radioed for help. Two men were arrested and tossed into a cruiser but bolted while the police were dealing with the other rowdies. (*Toronto Star*, September 12, 1985)

The oscillations between perceiving behavior as drunken folly and perceiving it as behavior with serious consequences probably in part explain moral ambivalence toward drinking and drunken behavior, including the aggression and violence linked to the use of alcohol. I will give several illustrations of this type of contextual framework change, as part of what could be called a naturalistic framing experiment.

The more detailed behavioral aspects of drunken driving are not as salient to the public eye as are those of drunken aggression. This is probably in part due to the fact that the serious consequences of impaired driving tend to overshadow any other aspects of alcohol-influenced behavior exhibited by a drunken driver. In addition (and more importantly for the present discussion), drunken aggression is typically preceded by interactional sequences and occurs in the open, as opposed to the drunken driver's relatively solitary presence in the front seat of a car. It is much more visible to outsiders. If we focus exclusively on the behavioral level without regard to potential consequences and moral implications, even behavior exhibited in connection with drunken driving is amenable to comic framing. Consider the following news item, which in itself, stripped of its framing possibilities, would not seem to warrant mass media attention:

> The man came driving at a snail's pace down the middle of the three-lane highway 87.
>
> A police patrol from Sollefteå became suspicious.
>
> The man did not react when the police used stop signals or honked their horns.
>
> After a while one policeman stepped out of his car and caught up with the strange vehicle on foot. He knocked on the windshield and on the side window.
>
> Still no reaction. The driver stared stiffly straight ahead with his hands holding the steering wheel in a cramped way.

> As a last resort the police barricaded the road with their car. They parked it about 10 meters in front of the slowly approaching vehicle.
>
> The man drove straight into the police car. He backed off and took another run—and rammed the police car a second time.
>
> At long last the policemen got the helplessly intoxicated driver out of his car. All attempts at interrogating the drunken driver were fruitless. (*Expressen*, Stockholm, Sweden, June 16, 1985; my translation)

We have here an undeniable comic effect (and no doubt this aspect of the story was what led to its publication). At the same time, the depicted event was serious enough: The driver's behavior was highly dangerous for the policemen in their car, and potentially so for other individuals who might have happened to be on the road in his vicinity. As for readers' reactions, the incident is no doubt viewed seriously by many of the same people who cannot help finding it funny. The ambiguity is there, and so is the moral ambivalence. A typical reaction in the face of such basic ambiguity is to shake our heads while laughing or smiling.

Wherein lies the possibility of viewing the above-described sequence of actions comically, as an instance of human folly? Or, to put it differently, what are some of the factors that determine such a comic framing? A possible (but no doubt only partial) answer is provided by Erving Goffman's analysis of the comic impact of some types of behavior. He cites Henri Bergson's thoughts on the matter: "Any arrangement of acts and events is comic which gives us, in a single combination, the illusion of life and the distinct impression of a mechanical arrangement" (Bergson, 1911, p. 69; as cited in Goffman, 1974, p. 38). In the behavior of the drunken driver described above, there is an ambiguity or tension between (1) a "guided doing," to use Goffman's terminology, in a purposive social framework; and (2) an externally determined physical occurrence, rather like some phenomenon in the natural sciences. (These are of course instances of a more general "conceptual dyad" [see, e.g., Nisbett, 1976] in the framing of behavior, which is familiar from the philosophy of science: the causal vs. the teleological.) The man appears to have been suspended between the two explanatory realms of physical/pharmacological determination and (more or less rational) goal-directed behavior. His conduct at the wheel suggested the automatism of a natural object. At the same time he was *driving* a car, and for such an activity there are no purely pharmacological and physiological determinants in sight. Instead, it has to be attributed to goal-directedness, albeit of a rather pathetic nature.

Sometimes the opposite happens: Presumably inanimate objects display salient aspects of guidedness. This results in the same ambiguity and humorous effect. Who doesn't find a robot funny, especially if it is equipped with extremities resembling arms, legs, and head? Cognitive structuring principles underlying this fact are exploited by break dancers and by comedians acting like robots, dolls, or mannequins—and robots acting like comedians or break dancers would probably be equally funny. Note also that some comedians (e.g., W. C. Fields, Dean Martin) have made a career out of mimicking drunks. Bergson's "illusion of life and the distinct impression of a mechanical arrangement" are present in all such behaviors and in the scenarios that make up their social context.

Social and moral contexts more serious than those associated with the production and consumption of newspaper texts do not totally rule out the possibilities of comic framing of alcohol-related behavior and the verbal acknowledgments of such (even by persons in very consequential social roles):

> A drinker who decided to go for a middle-of-the-night joy ride in a $200,000 harbour tour boat has been sentenced to 60 days in jail.
>
> "When he steals he sure picks a good one, doesn't he?" District Court Judge Hugh O'Connell commented yesterday. He also placed Ronald Daniel Floyd on probation for a year. (*Toronto Star*, October 16, 1987)

Even when the consequences of the drinking person's acts are extremely serious in terms of both material costs and human injuries, the possibilities of humorous framings aided by causally ambiguous and socially ambivalent thematic cues persist. A comical framing is reflected in the headline "Drug-Crazed Driver Was One-Man Wrecking Crew" (implying rational but in this context mistaken guidedness) and underscored by the final interaction related in the following excerpt:

> Half-crazed with drugs and booze, Mark Charles Cowling climbed into his car and drove down Kingston Rd. at high speed, weaving through traffic and hopping from lane to lane.
>
> Near Woodbine Ave. he rammed the back of another car and forced it into a hydro pole. Soon afterwards he rear-ended another car and sent it off the road.
>
> Cowling still wasn't finished. He picked up speed again, swerved into the passing lane and smashed into the rear of a third car, whose driver lost control.
>
> Then he hit a motorcycle so hard that it leaped into the air and landed on the roof of the car ahead. The driver and passenger, who was six months pregnant, were sent flying.
>
> After leaving a long trail of destruction and three people lying injured last Oct. 4, Cowling bit the policeman who arrested him. . . . (*Toronto Star*, May 4, 1983)

Similarly, in the case of a man who drove a bulldozer "through houses, barns, trees and a truck" in rural Alberta, the only comment by either the driver or his companion (who were both drunk on "white lightning") that was cited in a terse news item of 100 words or so was this: "That got us good and stoned" (*Toronto Star* [CP], October 8, 1981). Other types of comments made by the participants would no doubt have been abundantly available for an unambiguously serious framing of the incident. Apparently, the comment was selected primarily to reflect a comic framing of alcohol-induced reality, in tune with our alternation between different perceptions of its etiology and our consequent ambiguous attitudes toward even dangerous drunken behavior.

In this manner, serious occurrences of interpersonal violence or threats of such during drinking provide us with the same kind of material for comedy-enhancing etiological ambiguities as other types of intoxicated behavior. Framing an action by putting it in the context of role expectations applied to the elderly and the handicapped (and thus specifying the nature of the guided behavior normally to be expected) helps in making the following story titillatingly ambiguous enough to warrant a fairly prominent spot in a major evening newspaper:

> A drunken pensioner in a wheelchair has created a fracas in a senior citizens' home in Lidköping.
>
> In a totally reckless manner he drove around in the home firing shots with a pistol.
>
> The staff [members] were threatened with a knife. . . .
>
> The incident occurred last fall and has now been brought to court. The pensioner has been charged with illegal possession of a firearm and criminal threats.
>
> He confessed to having been intoxicated, but did not agree that he had threatened anybody. The pistol he just used to shoot blanks and to frighten away uninvited guests, he said. . . . (*Aftonbladet*, Stockholm, Sweden, February 28, 1985; my translation)

(The patient's ambulating in a wheelchair may have vaguely added to the cues implying natural determination.)

Even in the serious context of domestic violence, or violence between a man and a woman in general, ambiguity in framing is inherent when connected to alcohol use. In the following excerpt, the comic framing (indicated by the headline "Woman in Bar Fight with Former Champ Had 'Great Left Hook'") is aided by the celebrity status of one of the participants, by the nature of his claim to fame, and by the role-discordant behavior of the female participant:

> Former heavyweight boxing champion Leon Spinks was involved in a fist fight with a woman at a Las Vegas night club Monday and was escorted from the tavern by officers, police said. According to police Spinks was led from Botany's Restaurant on East Flamingo Road after the 5:15 a.m. incident. No charges were filed. "It was between Leon and a woman," said Botany's general manager, Jeff Leopold. "The argument started because she wanted to leave, but Leon wanted to stay. He slapped her and she returned with punches, scoring well. She had a great left hook. He then took her to the ground and hit her a couple of times, then left." . . . (*Toronto Star*, April 17, 1985)

The expressions "scoring well" and "a great left hook" add to the reader's framing options and the ensuing ambiguity. Placing the episode within the context of a spectator sport, essentially a less than serious game, enhances the comical framing cues available.

In regard to drunken comportment, it is possible to see even oneself as a naturally determined phenomenon. It is easier to marvel (and laugh) at one's behavior when it is interchangeably seen as a natural phenomenon independent of consciously guided intent. When actions are seen solely as natural phenomena, on the other hand—as suggested by the terms "automatism," "split personality" patterns, "blackouts," and the like—they become just frightening.

Tavern violence, as noted earlier, has a special semiotic status in much of Western society. It also has special interactional dynamics, which are probably linked both to the effects of alcohol and to the social definitions and belief structure built up around it. The predictability that comes with such stereotyping makes the events of a saloon brawl seem containable and relatively harmless, and thus makes it easier for participating individuals to make light of it. This is especially true after the fact, when the events have been linguistically contained through typification and thus cognitively mastered (and, perhaps, when such typification can be expected to lessen social disapproval):

> STOWE, Vt. (UPI)—Oliver Reed, the burly British actor who has starred in such movies as The Four Musketeers, seems to be taking his swashbuckling roles seriously these days.
>
> The 43-year-old actor was arrested early yesterday on charges of disorderly conduct, unlawful mischief and simple assault following what Stowe police described as a bar fight.
>
> "This is the first time I've had to spend the whole night in jail," Reed said yesterday afternoon. The actor was released on $500 bail pending a court appearance today.
>
> He was reached at a bar up the road from The Pub at Stowe, where police said the brawl took place. Reed's response to the incident was lighthearted.

> "I'm not angry at anybody, I just think this is marvellous," said the actor, who had just finished filming Death Bite in Toronto, where in an interview with The Star's Lynda Hurst only last month, he denied the vivid tales about his alleged bad boy antics. . . . (*Toronto Star*, October 13, 1981)

The line between human folly on the one hand, and dangerous risk, violence, and crime on the other, is impossible to draw, since there is no common logical territory where they exist contiguously and where lines can be drawn; instead, there is an either–or oscillation *on the part of the observer*. Attempts at providing content to the framing ambiguity such as explaining what are basically variations and alternations in our perception of the occurrence by referring to characteristics of the objective phenomenon itself, seem to lead to "mystification." Through this process the phenomenon of drunken comportment itself, and distinctions between guided doings and natural determination, are blurred into a mysterious realm. This may also be a way of resolving the basic ambivalence in our moral orientation toward drunken behavior.[2]

Mystification is illustrated in an account of a spring celebration in Stockholm, Sweden. Under the headline "Famous Smile Provoked Holiday Celebrators," the story tells what happened when the neighbors of an apartment in central Stockholm were frightened by the sound of a gunshot at about noon on a Good Friday and called the police:

> When the first policemen arrived at the scene, a man on wavering feet was standing in the hall with a pistol tucked under his belt. The gun was taken away, and the man was handcuffed and taken out to police detective Sture Larsson in the police van, which was parked around the corner.
>
> No one was made any the wiser by this. For one thing, the man was not in a very conversational state, and whatever he said need not have been the truth.
>
> The questions asked were these: Are there other people in the apartment? Has anyone been injured? Are there other weapons inside? . . .
>
> A few ordinance police arrived at the scene and closed off the street. The one closest to me sighed. He was just at the end of his shift when this assignment came.

2. In addition to mystification, there are other solutions to this special form of cognitive dissonance that involve projecting and objectifying the observer's cognitive processes. One of these has been evident in some of the excerpts cited to this point: a paternalistic attitude in describing alcohol-related episodes and actors in these episodes. In such cases, the drinker's behavior is described indulgently, as a parent would describe a child's behavior. The inherent ambiguity of cognition is here not projected onto the occurrence or its actors and resolved somehow, as is done in mystification, but is focused on the writer and the reader. The latter is invited to join the writer in disposing of the ambiguity as just childish or juvenile, and thus not serious (or even real).

"Now I'll get bawled out when I get home."

More policemen arrived. Six of them had bulletproof vests, gas masks, and submachine guns. Now things were getting serious. The six men got ready and ran down the street, keeping close to the wall of the building, and went through the door into 43 Döbelnsgatan.

The rest of us stood quietly and listened. We could almost hear the thumps from the tear gas canisters, the shouts, and the rattle of the submachine guns.

But, actually, what we heard was the voice of police detective Sture Larsson, full of relief. Somebody at police headquarters had gotten through to the apartment on the phone. The two people inside had promised to open the door.

A few minutes later two tired and absent-looking men were sitting in the police van.

"Nobody that I know," said Sture Larsson.

The three men in the apartment at 43 Döbelnsgatan had apparently gotten into their Easter liquor and made an early start. Around noon on Good Friday, one of them seemed to have achieved a state where time and space ceased to exist. He had taken his gun and shot at a reproduction of Leonardo da Vinci's "Mona Lisa" that was hanging on the wall.

Now he was on his way to sober up, be interrogated, and probably be charged with illegal possession of a firearm and endangering public safety.

For the rest of us it was all over. (Arne Söderlund, *Dagens Nyheter*, Stockholm, Sweden, April 6, 1984; my translation)

This report of drunken behavior illustrates a commonly encountered reaction: the removal of the motivations and actions of the drunken person from the ordinary frameworks in which we structure our daily activities and concerns. It is effectively contrasted to the mundane concerns of the policemen on the scene. (The reader may have noted that the target of this inexplicable attack, the famous smile that has become an icon of human enigma, also strengthens the theme of mystical processes and motivations.) We are dealing with another reality, one in which everyday salience and reasoning are suspended. The nature of this state is sometimes indicated by mysterious or eerie language, such as when intoxication is referred to as being "zonked" or "spifflicated" (a slang term used in the 1920s; see Wentworth & Flexner, 1974). The currently rather popular "bombed," "stoned," "smashed," and "plastered" are designations that refer allegorically to occurrences in the realm of natural forces. By connotation they place drunkenness and related comportment in this sphere. Recent years have seen a shift in viewing many alcohol-related phenomena away from a "free will" perspective, and an inclusion of a growing number of these into the paradigms of natural science. There has been a parallel shift from the personal responsibility of the drinker (generally a guided being) to the substance of alcohol (always a natural substance) and to physiological factors residing within the drinker (cf. the recent discussion on the medical, legal, and moral status of alcoholism).[3]

Mystification of the ideation and motivation of a drunken person is sometimes even more clearly aided by the content of interaction:

> Staff Sergeant Jack Press of Metro police testified that [Russell Petten, 23,] and his friend Gary Blagdon, 21, of Wellesley St. E[ast], had been drinking in a Yonge St. tavern last March 10, where they met Norman McBain, 56, of Gerrard St. W[est]. They later took McBain to his home because he was intoxicated and sat in his apartment "talking about things that were evil," the officer said.
>
> One of the "evil" things was considered to be a bottle of vodka and they poured its contents down the toilet.
>
> McBain then produced two handguns, which also were considered evil, Press said.
>
> Blagdon took one of them and pointed it at Petten.
>
> "A struggle ensued and Petten got the gun away from Blagdon, handled it in a careless manner and Blagdon was shot in the chest," Press said.
>
> The bullet went through his heart. . . . (*Toronto Star*, February 2, 1980)

In addition to the tension between the consequentiality of the sober world and the nonconsequentiality of the serious drinker's world, the tension between guided doing and natural determination is evident in descriptions of a drinker's behavior that present us with the ambiguity of determinant cues, resulting in a comic framing. The style and tone of the report on the shooting of da Vinci's masterpiece admirably catch the ambiguity of framing, as well as the mystification that results from locating the ambiguity and alternation in characteristics of the *actors* and from trying to resolve it statically, instead of seeing it as a dynamic process in which the *observer's* structurings alternate. The ambiguity resides in the way we as observers perceive the phenomenon of drunken comportment; for the drinkers themselves, the juxtaposition of guided doing and natural determination does not exist. They experience phenomenological continuities where our conceptual apparatus assumes different realms.

3. An ambiguity in framing is perhaps reflected in expressions such as "half-stoned," "half-shot," "half-corned," and the like, by which one may be trying to solve the ambiguity by standing with one leg in the domain of natural forces.

Possible Cultural Limits of the Frameworks

I do not claim to have a clear conception of the cultural and geographic boundaries of the applicability of natural determination and human guidedness as a pair of structuring frameworks, or of temporal variations in their relevance. The point of introducing them through the appreciation of humor into the subject area of alcohol's connections with aggression and physical violence—an area that neither in its empirical nor in its moral dimensions would seem to have much room for humor and mirth—is that to the extent that this type of humor is widely appreciated in a cultural sphere, the cognitive and social principles on which they are based are probably also widely used to structure human actions and the social world generally. The use of humor is a good cross-cultural (and unobtrusive) test of prevalent structuring principles, since there exists an uncontaminated criterion: the appreciation or lack of appreciation of the specific type of humor.

No doubt the straightforward distinction between natural determination and guided doing is less applicable in cultures with pronounced animistic beliefs. In order to make it more general, without losing features of the distinction that are useful for present purposes, we should perhaps instead of "natural" determination (a conception colored by Western natural-scientific biases) speak of "foreign" or "alien" determination to cover interpretations of behavior in which the actor is seen as not himself/herself, but under the influence (!) of some foreign entity, such as a force or a spirit (!). It may be worth noting that animistic determination is used in some humorous depictions of behavior; it is often tacitly contrasted with guided doings of the regular kind. This type of humorous tension between animism and guided doing can be seen in children's shows such as *Fraggle Rock* (where, to our amusement, even a garbage pile shows guidedness in his/her/its behavior). *The Muppet Show*, *The Wizard of Oz*, and innumerable other presentations illustrate the same humor-producing tension.[4]

There are animistic interpretations of alcohol-related behavior: North American Indians, for example, when first introduced to alcohol, interpreted the alcohol-induced changes as caused by evil spirits (MacAndrew & Edgerton, 1969). Also, religious sects and shamans have

4. The closest thing to animism in modern society is perhaps a rigid, "inhuman" determination by behavior norms and rules—domination by external human agents or by rules foreign to the actor's real body and mind. It is exemplified by the behavior of a bureaucrat—a favorite target of humor in some European countries, at least. The connotations of terms such as "*apparat*chik" and "*techno*crat" are definitely mechanistic and causal.

used alcohol (and drugs) to invoke various spirits and forces. Some remnants of such beliefs and structurings seem to persist in our language for alcohol and its use; the old linguistic baggage includes the aforementioned "spirits" and "being under the influence," as well as concepts such as "demon rum" and "the devil in the bottle," which were used to make aspects of drunken comportment more understandable and more easily morally targeted.

On the whole, though, it seems that the conceptual phenomena underlying Goffman's distinction between guidedness and natural determination cover most of the explanations of human behavior, including drunken comportment. These two clusters support much of our current conceptual apparatus. In fact, the distinction is one of the cornerstones in constructing the world as experienced (and, which is largely the same thing, making it meaningful and predictable). One behaves very differently toward inanimate objects than toward other human beings (and if one did not, the guidedness of one's own doings would be questioned, with potentially very serious consequences). To treat someone as if he/she belongs in the natural frame really is to treat that individual as a "nonperson" (e.g., Goffman, 1961). (The consequences for social interaction of our implicit categorizations of intoxicated persons and their behavior are evident here. They deserve more focused attention than they will receive in this book.)

Tension between the Two Frameworks in Scientific Research

The discussion up to this point would be rather peripheral, were it not the case that the tension between perceiving drunken behavior as a natural phenomenon and perceiving it as goal-directed behavior is also richly evident in the current scientific approach to the relationship between alcohol and aggressive behavior. (The reason why researchers are not laughing at these phenomena is that they typically do not directly experience this inherent ambiguity through naturalistic observation of concrete episodes of alcohol-related behavior; they are more focused on the processing of aggregated data. Besides, there probably is a humorless "scientific frame" for observing phenomena.) To date it seems that the natural-level framework with mechanistic models of explanation, based largely on the identification of alcohol as a pharmacological agent that causes specific changes in physiological processes and identifiable psychological abilities, has had the upper hand. Key variants in this explanatory genre are the ideas that alcohol is a "disinhibitor," a "facilitator," a "trigger," or even a "catalyst" for aggressive behavior. Often these ideas remain on a vague conceptual level. More specific causal modelings refer to pharmacological effects of alcohol on the cellular level of the brain. Such models are commonly linked to psychodynamic notions:

> The effects of alcohol are not due to stimulation of the higher centers of the brain, but are due to the depression of those centers. First, the centers regulating conduct, judgment and self-criticism are depressed concurrently with those parts of the brain regulating the finer functions of co-ordination. Progressively the centers of basic emotional control are depressed, and the inhibitory functions of the centers are lost with an alteration in the conduct of the individual moving towards the "miserable, mean, nasty and brutish" as described by Hobbes. (Paul, 1975, p. 16)

The alternative explanatory framework, which invokes human guidedness, has its proponents mainly among social anthropologists and other social scientists. For these theorists, broad behavior themes, primarily those invoking the social functionality of some drunken behavior, provide scaffoldings for explanatory attempts. Perhaps the best-known of such thematic explanations is MacAndrew and Edgerton's (1969) explanation of drunken comportment. They view it as basically determined by social definitions of alcohol use occasions as "time out." More recently, Burns (1980) has presented a convincing description of the alcohol-related behavior of young men in a pub-crawling sequence in which their behavior shows the same guided, "within-limits" character as postulated by MacAndrew and Edgerton on the basis of a thorough review of the anthropological literature. Drunken behavior is here seen as rather exclusively determined in a basically instrumental fashion by socially provided behavior norms. Pharmacological effects of alcohol are downplayed. The same tendency is evident in microsociological treatises of drinking behavior, such as Cavan's (1966) otherwise laudable ethnographic study of public drinking places in San Francisco and Anderson's (1978) equally perceptive study of "Jelly's" in Chicago. As far as one can judge from their description, the patrons might as well have been drinking orange juice; all behavior is ascribed to normative and other social factors, without any attempt at examining whether alcohol's effects had any impact on concrete sequences of individual behavior and interaction, and (more centrally for the nomothetic aims of their studies) whether normative expectations had evolved on the basis of observed and experienced effects of alcohol.

Attempts at transcending the explanatory scaffoldings provided by guidedness and natural causality easily lead to mystification even in scientific explanations of intoxicated behavior. Such explanations often emanate from a structuralist base, and the ambiguities involved are not limited to the explanation of behavior after drinking. Explanatory concepts are introduced without a clear location in either of the major explanatory frameworks and without any explication of the determinant processes involved. Needless to say, descriptions of etiology do not make allowance for objective and phenomenal effects of alcohol. In this way the attitude toward the requirement of isomorphism in empirical processes and theoretical structurings is even laxer than in common social–thematic explanations. In some cases, there is not even a clear specification of the behavior to be explained. The causal processes referred to seem to be phenomenal or mentalistic in nature, and thus explanable in terms of individual behavior; at other times a version of a direct, almost "organic" influence by social, cultural, and/or historical factors is assumed. In the latter case, motivations, orientations, and actions of humans are left totally unspecified. The general lack of distinction between pre-empirical concept formation and the ambition to explain cultural phenomena and behavior linked to these is already evident in the works of the social structuralist par excellence, Lévi-Strauss, as has been pointed out by Burridge (1967) and several other authors before and after him. It is not my intention to deny the very important contributions made by social structuralists to the study of man and his culture. However, for the purpose of explaining drunken behavior, the structures of myth and thinking are not enough; in addition to this logical–conceptual framework we need complementary explanations of the determinant *processes* involved. This variety of potential explanations of drunken comportment however is not a concern of this book, since it is not a concept specific enough for a thorough analysis.

Common framings of human action thus also intrude on the conceptual givens that determine the scientist's basic categorizations and his/her universes of theoretical interest. As researchers, we ought to be more attentive to our boundedness by such general cognitive frameworks in our explanations of acts and events. The fact that every day we classify episodes and sequences of behavior into the goal-directed and the mechanically caused may make it hard for us to see actual etiological identities or similarities (as well as etiologically/causally significant differences) between different types of events and behavior sequences. This makes theoretical integration difficult. These considerations are important in the current theoretical stalemate in the explanation of drunken behavior. Neither an exclusive natural-level emphasis, nor a similar stress on human guidedness, nor nonanalytical mystification is an acceptable way out of the dilemma. For the time being, the best analytical strategy seems to be a return to the basics: looking at drunken behavior and interaction naturalistically, within their concrete individual and, above all, interactional sequences. In this way, the exclusiveness of the explanatory frames may be seen to be conceptual in origin, and attempts at theoretical integration are more likely to reflect the empirical integration found in real-life processes.

I hope that this book will to some extent help provide a balance between the two frameworks of human guidedness and inanimate causal determination, and that it will aid in some integrational attempts. In scientific explanations of behavior, there must be intrinsic linkages between the two realms; using them as exclusive, alternative frameworks for drunken comportment will not suffice. We must try to overcome this cognitive limitation. There are intimate interactions between the two frameworks as they are linked to alcohol use: the natural causality of the chemical substance and a drinker's guided orientations under its influence. An adequate theory of intoxicated behavior must take both of these into account and try to give each its proper due.

THE ORGANIZATION OF THE BOOK

The major focus in the chapters of this book that report findings from my empirical study is on the *outcomes*, the end products, of some of the pharmacological, psychological, social, symbolic, and interactional processes that increase the probability that an alcohol use occasion will involve aggressive behavior. The focus is on outcomes because the sampling units for the study consist of episodes of violence. The decision to concentrate on such episodes sets its own limits on the types of questions that can be asked and generalizations that can be made. (See Chapter 9 for a discussion of one central feature of such samples, which narrows the analytical possibilities.) Still, in the context of presently available research on naturally occurring aggression, the data presented here support an augmentation of questions asked and generalizations made possible. (As I have noted earlier, in later publications I hope to take a more direct look at determinant *processes* linking alcohol and aggression by means of analyses of other types of aggression episodes and of data from direct observation of intoxicated behavior.)

The main strength of these data is that they represent "real," naturally occurring events of aggression and violence. To a great extent, this circumvents the problems of external validation that characterize experimental studies on aggression: Ethical considerations in such studies closely confine the possibilities of manipulating the measures of aggression, and limiting "cover stories" are needed in order to avoid confounding influences from the subjects' discrepant definitions of the situation. Studying real-life aggression, albeit after the fact, makes it possible to sidestep this issue (at some cost), since this lets the whole instrumental and semiotic richness of human aggression into the data, and we can thus try to make sense of and explain it on a more general level. There are obvious weaknesses inherent in after-the-fact analyses of any phenomena; these hardly need expounding here, since they are readily available in textbooks on research methodology. The present data should be seen as a useful and probably necessary complement to more controlled approaches in the study of the connections between alcohol use and aggression. They are also a long-needed complement to the analyses of official documents of detected crimes of violence.

Where constellations of actors and settings are later analyzed with a mainly descriptive intent, it is my hope that these will contribute to a social ecology of aggression episodes and specifically of alcohol-related aggression. There is a definite need for descriptive analyses of real-life aggression episodes that can serve as models for controlled studies of aggression and can provide information on their prevalence and incidence in general populations and their subpopulations. Both middle-range data and middle-range theories have been missing in the study of human aggression. With the social-psychological interest and the interactional and transactional focus in the recent study of human aggression and violence (see, e.g., Campbell & Gibbs, 1986), this is being rectified. Considering the high prevalence of alcohol use in connection with serious aggression, studies of the role of alcohol along these communicational dimensions are needed. The empirical approach presented here is part of a first attempt.

After this first introductory chapter, which has touched on the broadest of conceptual issues related to the explanation of intoxicated behavior, Chapter 2 reviews the most important types of studies that have been conducted with the purpose of testing the existence or estimating the strength of the relationship between alcohol and violence in society.

The rationale and fieldwork for the survey of residents in the Canadian community are described in Chapter 3. The representativeness of the final interview sample obtained is assessed in this chapter. The reader is referred to Appendix A for a more detailed discussion of methodological issues; for information on "crucial survey conditions" (Kish, 1965); and for a description of the interview situation, which together with the questions asked makes up the "measuring instrument" in this type of survey research. Items from the questionnaire that are relevant for the subject matter of the book are presented in Appendix B. The risk of social desirability effects is especially acute with questions on the respondents' alcohol use and experiences of aggression and violence, the two central clusters of variables in this study. Validity issues linked to these are also discussed in Appendix A (which should essentially be seen as part of Chapter 3). In this chapter, a 1-year census taken of all the violent crimes recorded by the police during a period running concurrently with the fieldwork for the interview survey is also described.

Chapter 4 focuses on aggression experienced during a 1-year period by adults living in the city. Using the past 12 months as a reference period makes it possible to estimate the prevalence and incidence of victimization in physical violence and in threats of such violence. The main focus is on the relationship between gender and age and the risk of victimization, but the alcohol use patterns of community residents are also briefly related to victimization experiences. In addition, witnessing of physical violence and the prevalence of this experience in subgroups of the population are described. A comparison between the interview data and the census of violent crimes allows estimates of "dark figures" (proportions of violence that did not come to the attention of the police) for central population groups.

The analysis of specific episodes of physical violence, which constitutes the main focus of the remainder of the book, begins in Chapter 5. Parallel descriptive analyses are carried out on the reported episodes of violent crime in the community and the most recent violent victimizations of survey respondents, although major differences in sampling procedures make these comparisons very tentative. In this chapter the nature of the episodes is described, without yet introducing alcohol use as a factor.

The statistical role of alcohol use is introduced in the analysis of the violence episodes in Chapter 6. The analyses are generally of the conventional type found in research on the role of alcohol in violent crime, but the systematic nature of the interview data allows a closer look at characteristics of the participants and settings, as well as at their relationship to the probability of alcohol's presence in the episode.

In Chapter 7, the characteristics of participating individuals and the settings are examined in relation to the types of violent acts committed by the assailants. The extent to which alcohol use by assailants and victims determines what acts will be used is a central question and is addressed here. Special analyses are made of the extent to which alcohol use leads to the indiscriminate use of different types of violent acts.

Chapter 8 brings us to the consequences of the violent episodes in terms of physical injury and medical activity. The patterning of these consequences is used to further test the hypothesis that alcohol leads to a more indiscriminate use of violence and generally to an exacerbation of violence. (Regrettably, it was not possible to get information about injuries, medical attention, incidents that went to court, etc., for violent crimes recorded by the police. As a consequence, factors influencing these outcomes could not be investigated for these episodes of violent crime, in a way parallel to the study of violent events accessed through interviews with community residents.)

Finally, Chapter 9 summarizes the main findings of the study and puts these in a broad theoretical perspective. Much of the theoretical impetus is gained from these findings, but the discussion ranges beyond the scope of the data of this study. Here I also return to the pre-empirical and metatheoretical questions that have been introduced in the present chapter. The theoretical relevance of the findings is rather general, and the theoretical conclusions primarily take the form of an agenda for the future.

2

Studies of the Role of Alcohol in Real-Life Violence

STUDIES OF ALCOHOL INVOLVEMENT IN OFFICIALLY DOCUMENTED VIOLENCE

It has almost exclusively been left up to studies of crime that has come to the attention of the police or has been processed in the courts to provide quantitative information on the aggregated role of alcohol in naturally occurring aggressive encounters.[1] There are numerous studies based on officially documented violence in the published literature (see Pernanen, 1976; Roizen & Schneberk, 1977; and Wolfgang, 1958, for reviews of many of these). In Table 2.1, findings from some fairly representative studies in this genre from different parts of the world are summarized. Only studies in which information on alcohol use was reported for both the offenders and the victims are included.

1. The designations "real-life" and "naturally occurring" are used in order to exclude consideration of the aggression or violence that takes place in experimental settings where alcohol consumption is one of the independent variables manipulated. This also rules out the quasi-experimental study of alcohol's connection with aggression in contrived party settings (e.g., Boyatzis, 1974, 1975). Observational studies in real-life settings have not focused on aggressive behavior systematically enough to allow even the most rudimentary generalizations, and so these studies are not discussed here either. Empirical and theoretical issues related to these types of studies will be discussed in the upcoming monograph mentioned in Chapter 1 (footnote 1).

The North American data pertain mostly to homicides. Relatively low rates of homicides (and thus a relative dearth of study material) steer Scandinavian studies toward the exploration of the role of alcohol in nonfatal assaults. The published data on alcohol involvement in rapes and robberies are very scattered as to time, location, and methods used. They are not presented in the table, both because they present a very confusing array of alcohol involvement proportions and because they are of somewhat less relevance for the empirical material presented in this book. The most ambitious North American studies to date reporting on the role of alcohol in rapes and robberies are Amir's (1971) for rapes and Normandeau's (1968) for robberies. In the former study, 24% of offenders and 31% of victims ($n = 646$) had been drinking prior to the rapes. In Normandeau's sample of police reports on robberies, by contrast, drinking by both offenders (7%) and victims (12%) was low ($n = 892$). A Canadian study of homicides reported to the police found that about 20% of offenders in robberies that led to homicides had been drinking, while 11% of victims in these robbery murders had been drinking ($n = 190$; Statistics Canada, 1976). By contrast, in both Poland (Marek, Widacki, & Hanausek, 1974) and Finland (Leppä, 1974), drinking by robbery victims was close to 70%, as determined from police reports. This points to considerable differences in violent crime patterns (and no doubt in record keeping as well) between different countries.

Table 2.1 shows drinking by offenders and victims separately. Another common statistic is the *total* alcohol involvement in the crime occurrences, which is the percentage of episodes in which either the offender or the victim or both had been drinking prior to the episode (i.e., alcohol had been used by at least one of the two principal actors). When these "impact figures" are sufficiently striking, as when they reach the 50–60% level, caution seems to be thrown to the winds and they are seen as reflections of the true *causal* contribution of alcohol use to the level of violent crime. The most thorough of North American studies presenting this statistic was carried out on police reports and autopsy reports of criminal homicide in Philadelphia between 1948 and 1952 (Wolfgang, 1958). It found a total alcohol involvement of 64%.

Despite an increase in the prevalence of other psychoactive drug use in the general population and especially in populations at high risk of violent crime during the last couple of decades (e.g., Haberman & Baden, 1978), more recent American reports still find that alcohol is implicated in a great proportion of homicides. Thus, in autopsies performed on 4,092 victims of criminal homicide in Los Angeles during the 1970–79 period, alcohol was detected in the blood of 46% of these

TABLE 2.1. Drinking by Offenders and Victims Prior to Assaults and Homicides, as Found in Studies Based on Police Reports and Court Records of Violent Crime and on Autopsies of Homicide Victims

			Offenders		Victims	
Author(s)	Location	Source of data	Sample *n*	% with alcohol present	Sample *n*	% with alcohol present
		Assaults				
Pittman & Handy (1964)	St. Louis, USA	Police reports	237	24%	241	25%
President's Commission on Crime in the District of Columbia (1966)	Washington, DC, USA	Police reports	121	35%	131	46%
Aho (1976)	Finland	Police reports	527	72%	527	45%
Wasikhongo (1976)	Mombasa, Kenya	Police reports	268	58%	251	58%
Wikström (1980)	Gävle, Sweden	Police reports	808	75%	754	54%
		Homicides				
Wolfgang (1958)	Philadelphia, USA	Police reports, autopsies	621	55%	588	53%
Criminal Justice Commission (1967)	Baltimore, USA	Police reports, autopsies	624	36%	578	47%
Verkko (1951)	Vyborg County, Finland	Court records	543	55%	543	48%
Virkkunen (1974)	Helsinki, Finland	Police reports, autopsies	114	66%	116	68%
Somander (1979)	Sweden	Court records, autopsies	99	70%	103	47%

victims (Goodman et al., 1986). The same approximate magnitude (42%) was found in autopsies of criminal homicide victims in Erie County, N.Y., for the period 1973–1983 (*n* = 792; Welte & Abel, 1985; see also Abel & Zeidenberg, 1985). This can be compared to the 53% reported by Wolfgang (1958) for Philadelphia about 25–30 years earlier (Table 2.1).

In the country of the present book's empirical study, Canada, the efforts of Guy Tardif should be mentioned in particular. On the basis of analyses of police reports, Tardif calculated levels of alcohol involvement from samples of the four major types of violent crimes committed in the city of Montreal during 1964 (Tardif, 1966, 1967). He found the following percentages (sample *n*'s in parentheses): rape victims, 16% (112); rape offenders, 31% (67); robbery victims, 16% (212); robbery offenders, 12% (117); assault victims, 25% (140); assault offenders, 37% (124); homicide victims, 22% (59); and homicide offenders, 28% (53). Statistics Canada, as noted earlier, conducted an analysis of all homicides in Canada during 1961–1974 (Statistics Canada, 1976) and found that 41% of these homicides were alcohol-related (*n* = 3,615). In addition, another 3% were either alcohol- or drug-related, with only a small proportion related to drug use alone; this puts the total alcohol involvement at about 44%. Gerson and Preston (1979) conducted a full census of aggressive behavior that came to the attention of the police during a 1-year period in an Ontario municipality. They found that 33% (*n* = 5,178) of these incidents were alcohol-related. However, among these incidents were included a number of threat episodes. If these are deleted and the alcohol involvement in physical violence recalculated, the proportion increases to 38% (*n* = 4,032).

The Scandinavian countries, with the possible exception of Denmark, show extremely high levels of alcohol involvement in homicides and assaults. A Danish study showed that the total alcohol involvement in criminal homicides between 1946 and 1970 was relatively low, 34% (Hansen, 1977). However, Finnish studies consistently reach levels of 55–75% (e.g., Aho, 1967, 1976; Verkko, 1951; Virkkunen, 1974). Norwegian studies show alcohol involvements in criminal violence of the same magnitude (Fekjaer, 1985; Bödal, 1987). A study from Iceland reports an alcohol involvement of 77% in homicides occurring during the period 1946–1970 (Hansen & Bjarnarson, 1974). The highest proportions, however, are reported in the literature on Swedish assaults and homicides, with figures consistently above 80% for total alcohol involvement (Kühlhorn, 1984; Somander, 1979; Wikström, 1985). In addition, a Swedish study on offenders found guilty of interpersonal crimes of violence and referred for forensic psychiatric examinations found that these individuals had been drinking in 68% of the crime episodes (Roslund & Larson, 1979). It is also interesting to note that in Greenland, where homicide rates have increased 13-fold between the late 1940s and the beginning of the 1980s, the total alcohol involvement in homicides for this period was 78% ($n = 92$), and homicide attempts in the late 1970s had an alcohol involvement figure of 97% ($n = 59$; Hansen, 1985). The high Scandinavian figures can no doubt in part be explained by Scandinavian officials' and researchers' greater sensitization to alcohol problems in general and to the presence of alcohol in violent crimes in particular. This assumption also implies that the figures for some other countries may to some extent underestimate the true alcohol involvement in violent crimes.

Studies from several other countries show the same type of pattern of alcohol involvement. In Table 2.1 I have, in addition to American and Scandinavian data, shown one set of figures from Kenya; this study and studies in Australia (76%; Bowden, Wilson, & Turner, 1958), South Africa (64%; Le Roux & Smith, 1964), France (76%; Verhaege & Schodet, 1959), and Austria (46%; Schumacher, 1923) present high proportions of drinking *victims* in homicides and assaults. The total alcohol involvement would in these cases have been even higher, considering the general tendency for offenders to have been drinking to a larger extent than victims, and the less than total correspondence between drinking by offenders and drinking by victims in the same episode.

RESEARCH APPROACHES WITH AGGREGATED DATA

However, all these convincing percentages must be related to relevant population figures so that we can arrive at standardized rates related to alcohol consumption (and have a great number of potential confounding variables controlled for in this way). None of the studies reporting on the prevalence of an alcohol component in violent crime have in fact related their findings to population bases or alcohol consumption rates, which would provide better comparability between the estimates of the studies. I have undertaken some calculations on homicide rates in Canada and Finland for 1974, which is the most recent year for which national data for alcohol involvement exist for both countries (Statistics Canada, 1976; Aho, 1976; Pernanen, 1989a). The homicide rates in the two countries are traditionally fairly similar; in 1974 they were 2.4 per 100,000 population in Canada and 2.3 in Finland. When rates were calculated separately for alcohol-related and alcohol-free homicide incidents on the basis of the best estimates available, the following rates were obtained:

	Canada	Finland
Alcohol	1.1	1.5
No alcohol	1.3	0.8
Total	2.4	2.3

When these figures were related to total sales of alcohol in the country, it became clear that the probability of an alcohol-related homicide per volume of alcohol sold was over 80% higher in Finland than in Canada. Several countries in southern Europe would show a much higher volume of alcohol consumed per alcohol-related homicide; this is evident from the low rates of homicides and the high rates of per capita alcohol consumption. Calculations of the type exemplified above are not possible for these countries, however, because of a lack of statistical information on the presence of alcohol in homicide cases.

The calculations above illustrate the limitations of the available percentage figures on alcohol involvement, which until recently have been the almost exclusive basis for establishing the existence and estimating the "real-life" strength of the relationship between alcohol use and violence. By tacit extension, they have often been interpreted as showing a direct relationship between the use of alcohol and the occurrence of aggressive behavior generally. Because of their bivariate nature they seem to invite rather simplistic explanations, in which suitable labels are invented for the substance of alcohol and its drinkers, and then given a quasi-explanatory status. Such is the case with the presumed "disinhibiting" or "catalytic" property of alcohol in bringing about violence, and the presumed trait or process of "disinhibition" in the person who has been drinking.

Another type of research approach is to look at the relationship between aggregated data on alcohol consumption in a population and the rates of violent crime. This method neutralizes the problem with population bases, since it deals with rates per population unit. However, because of the difficulties inherent in cross-national comparisons, the analyses of such data are usually restricted to time series analyses. Even a crude visual inspection of graphic representations of per capita consumption rates and rates of both homicides and assaults for Sweden during the 1856–1985 period indicates a fairly close relationship (although trend effects have not been controlled for, and the curves clearly diverge after the end of the 1970s; Central Bureau of Statistics, Sweden, 1987). On the other hand, a similar inspection of rates of homicides and assaults and per capita alcohol consumption in Ontario, Canada, for the period 1933–1972 showed very divergent trends (Carsjö, 1977). However, the more sophisticated analyses carried out to date generally point toward a fairly close connection between changes in alcohol consumption rates and changes in violent crime rates in the Scandinavian countries (Lenke, 1982; Skog, 1987).

Even this type of connection seems to be conditional on some other societal factors' being present, though. The determinant strength of aggregated alcohol consumption varied markedly among different societies in a four-country comparison, notably between Finland (where there was a strong effect of alcohol on the extent of violent crime) and France (where there was practically no effect), with Sweden and Denmark showing intermediate effects (Lenke, 1989). Causal processes underlying the aggregate-level relationship are thus more complicated than a mere bivariate connection between rates of alcohol use and rates of violence. This has been shown to be the case for Finland by Aho (1976) in a time trend study, in which he carried out a joint analysis of alcohol involvement percentages, rates of alcohol consumption, and rates of violent crime. If we were to assume that levels of alcohol consumption in a country are causally linked to levels of homicide, we would expect significant increases in alcohol consumption to be correlated not just with general increases in violent crime, but specifically with increases in *alcohol-related* violent crime. However, despite a major increase in per capita alcohol consumption in Finland during the years 1956–1974 and an increase in rates of violent crime, there was no increase in the total alcohol involvement of the violent crimes. On the other hand, Skog (1986) has shown in sophisticated time trend analyses of Norwegian data for the period 1951–1980 that the development in per capita alcohol consumption had a substantial impact on the number of deaths from all violent causes among men; he has demonstrated a similar effect on convictions for crimes of violence during the 1930–1982 period (Skog, 1987).

Police records of crimes of violence have also been used to assess the "natural experiments" provided through sudden decreases in the availability of alcoholic beverages, such as the closing of liquor outlets through strikes by liquor store employees (e.g., Takala, 1973); Saturday closings of such stores (Olsson & Wikström, 1982); and rationing of alcohol purchases or significant price increases (Lenke, 1982). These "experiments" may involve increases as well as decreases in availability, such as the opening of alcohol outlets in formerly "dry" areas or a marked increase in the number of outlets (Lenke, 1982), and lowering of the legal drinking age. The studies of decreased availability generally show distinct decreases in violent crime and domestic disturbances, as well as in injuries from different causes presenting at emergency rooms of hospitals (e.g., Karaharju & Stjernvall, 1974). Studies examining the effects of increased availability generally find increases in these factors. Such an effect was detected even in the present survey data from a Canadian community (Pernanen, 1989b).

PROBLEMS WITH USING POLICE AND COURT RECORDS

The relative ease with which police report data and court records can be subjected to analyses probably explains their widespread use. If knowing the proportional involvement of alcohol were our only research objective, and if we could safely assume that the incidents appearing in the police records were an unbiased sample of all violent incidents within the jurisdictional and geographical boundaries of our study, the use of police records would suffice for many purposes. However, although crimes known to the police are generally regarded as being the least biased source of continually and systematically recorded violent crimes, they are still far from totally unbiased. Even the best data sets of detected violent crimes are often biased as a result of factors that are idiosyncratic to the jurisdiction in which they were collected, such as police procedures and recording, area containment practices, clearance rates, and the like. Variations in these factors affect findings on the characteristics of the violent incidents and of the offenders and victims, and in all likelihood findings on the role of alcohol as well.

As is the case with most other forms of behavior that fall within the legal definitions of "crimes," the occurrences of interpersonal violence that come to the attention of the police form only a small part of the actual prevalence of interpersonal violence in any society (e.g., Aromaa, 1977b; Biderman, Johnson, McIntyre, & Weir, 1967; Central Bureau of Statistics, Sweden, 1981; Christie, Andenaes, & Skirbekk, 1965; Ennis, 1967; Evans & Leger, 1979; Hood & Sparks, 1974; Reiss, 1967; Solicitor General, Canada, 1983, 1984; U.S. Department of Justice, 1977; Wolfgang & Singer, 1978). The estimates of the ratio of undetected criminal violence to all criminal violence differ, but the ratio is substantial in the various jurisdictions in which it has been calculated. Only homicides have a detection rate that is close to unity in many jurisdictions. (As we shall see later, one of the findings of the present study is that the proportion of interpersonal violence reported to the community police was about 4%. However, the criteria for this study were set to include relatively mild forms of violence.)

If the results of analyses of police or court records are intended to provide estimates of the patterns of violent behavior in a jurisdiction, we have to take into account that the "dark figures" (i.e., proportions of unreported incidents) in interpersonal violence are not independent of central characteristics of violent episodes and the persons involved in these; they covary with some central factors. Numerous studies that have compared recorded crimes with general population surveys of the prevalence of criminal episodes have shown that, for instance, family violence is underrepresented to a disproportionate degree. This is also the case for violence among youths and in subgroups of the population with relatively high rates of criminality (e.g., Hood & Sparks, 1974; McClintock, 1963; Wikström, 1985). Other, more inferential indicators, such as characteristics of crimes in which a person other than the victim reported the event to the police or characteristics of refusals to press charges or testify in court, indicate the same pattern of bias. Generally, it can be said that violence in family or peer groups and in relatively self-contained (often criminally active) subcultures is underrepresented. Officially recorded crime incidents are thus not random or representative samples of the violent events that occur in a jurisdiction and that can be labeled "violent crimes" according to the criteria of the police or courts of justice.

By no means all perpetrators of detected violent crimes are caught or identified. Consequently, a further shortcoming of police records is the lack of information on offenders in a considerable proportion of known crime events. The clearance rate for violent crimes is much higher than for crimes against property; still, a considerable proportion of reports on violent crimes include only the scantiest information on the perpetrators, since their identity was not known to the victims or any witnesses, or they were not identified later on the basis of other evidence. Therefore, surveys carried out on, for example, prison populations, which are of great value for many other purposes, have passed through additional selective and biasing processes and cannot unquestioningly be accepted as estimates of the true role of alcohol in the violence that occurs in society.

In addition to the other factors mentioned, intoxicated offenders and especially known abusers of alcohol are more easily caught by police (Pernanen, 1981a). Alcohol abusers tend to be recidivists and thus often receive stiffer penalties (although in less serious crimes they may also be more generally diverted into treatment programs); thus, they populate prisons in greater proportions and for longer periods of time, and influence any estimates through these selection biases. With the additional cautionary remark that—depending on the nature of culturally and institutionally grounded semiotics of alcohol use and alcohol abuse in the particular jurisdiction involved—intoxication at the time of the violence can be used to disclaim responsibility both in courts and in survey responses, I only mention some results from one ambitious prison study. Roizen and Schneberk (1977) reanalyzed data collected by the U.S. Department of Justice (1975) and found high alcohol involvement figures not only for offenders in violent crimes, but also for offenders in property crimes. The percentages of drinking offenders were, for murders, 53% (n = 10,811); attempted murders, 48% (n = 2,088); manslaughter, 55% (n = 4,260); aggravated assault, 62% (n = 3,311); assault (simple and undetermined) 59% (n = 1,781); robbery with weapon, 39% (n = 11,113), and robbery without weapon, 41% (n = 5,504). There was also a tendency for recidivating offenders to have higher than average proportions of drinking at the time of the offense.

Even when information about offenders exists, police reports and court records do not include data on a number of potentially important determinants. Most importantly for present purposes, they often do not include any information, or specific enough information, on the nature of "alcohol use prior to the crime." Very little is known about amounts consumed, states of drunkenness, lengths of drinking episodes prior to the crime, types of beverage consumed, or the like in violent crime. It is safe to assume that many variables highly relevant to the explanation of why violence occurred have not been included in the great majority of occurrence reports. One consequence is that experimental studies of the influence of alcohol use on aggression have had no population basis to stand on. Only bare estimates of alcohol involvement have been available, and these are of no help in selecting alcohol use variables and the range of variation within these variables to guide systematic manipulation in experiments. Moreover, the samples obtained through official records of violent incidents are also biased against less severe violence occurring in the general population (Skogan, 1977), and their usefulness for a strategic integration with other methodologies for studying the relationship between alcohol use and aggression is therefore limited.

VICTIMIZATION SURVEYS

In order to overcome some of these weaknesses and to estimate the biases present in official records of violence, criminological, sociological, and statistically oriented studies have examined the prevalence of serious violence by means of the "victimization survey" method. In these studies, samples of individuals from the general population are asked how often they have been the victims of violence during a delimited reference period (e.g., the 12 months preceding the interview date). The major aim is to provide data on the true extent of different types of crimes, and to estimate the proportion of crime which does not come to the attention of the police. The aggression incidents asked about are (with some difficulty) restricted to what fits the definition of a violent crime: an assault, a rape or attempted rape, a robbery or attempted robbery, and so forth. Within this objective, it is natural that no less severe forms of aggression are asked about. For more theoretically oriented analyses, however, it would also be desirable to obtain data on subcriminal incidents of aggression (and the role of alcohol in these).

One important advantage of victimization surveys is that information is gathered specifically for systematic analyses. Questions are asked in a systematic and structured fashion, and not left up to the idiosyncratic procedures of different jurisdictions and of different officials recording information on crime episodes. Ideally, victimization surveys should also provide information that is missed because many violence episodes are not reported to the police. Still, there will be some missing information, especially on perpetrators of the criminal acts. In these cases, we encounter the same problem of missing data as caused by the less than total identification/apprehension rate in police data.

Since the primary aim of victimization studies is to arrive at better estimates of criminality of different kinds, many characteristics of the events of violence that are not directly linked to the administration of justice are disregarded or scantily investigated. To date no victimization studies have, to my knowledge, recorded the extent to which alcohol was used by one or more participants in criminal incidents.

In some important respects, the survey to be reported in the remainder of this book is a victimization study. It differs from earlier such studies in its greater emphasis on specific episodes, its focus on several types of aggression and on angry arousal, its detailed data on alcohol use events, and its role as one "leg" in a triangulation approach using observations in public drinking establishments and analyses of police records as complementary data sources. This book is mainly concerned with episodes of physical violence that have been made available both through interviews and through the routine record keeping of the police. Some illustrative material is also brought in from the observations carried out in public drinking establishments.

Victimization surveys also have some other potential shortcomings. The sampling frame is often such that subsegments of the populace most likely to be victimized by violent crime (criminal and alcoholic subgroups, slum dwellers, etc.) are underrepresented in the study, whether the sampling is based on an area frame or on population records (Pernanen, 1974; Wilson, 1981). Questions regarding occurrences of violence have to be retrospective, sometimes ranging over the adult life span of the respondent, and typically at least covering the most recent

12-month period. The problems with recall of different types of life events even for less ambitious reference periods have been well documented. Faulty recall can lead to underestimations and biases, in that some types of episodes are better remembered than other types. Under- or over-estimations due to forward or backward "telescoping" (i.e., mistakenly placing an event inside or outside the reference period) also have to be taken into account (Wolfgang & Singer, 1978). Finally, respondents may be reluctant to report violent events to an interviewer conducting a victimization survey, partly for the same reasons as those described above for underreporting of violent events to the police. In short, many of the same types of biases are at work as in studies of official records of crime, but interviews with the general population are still an important complement to such studies. Some of these problems are discussed in the next chapter and in Appendix A, where the methodology and fieldwork of the interview survey are described.

3

The Study of Alcohol Use and Aggression in a Canadian Community: Rationale, Methodology, and Fieldwork

In Chapters 4 to 8, I present findings from an intensive study of the prevalence of aggressive behavior and its concomitants among the residents of a community in northwestern Ontario, Canada. The main emphasis of the study was on the elucidation of the relationship between alcohol use and aggression. In this book, the main concern is with alcohol's connections with physical aggression; the relationship of violent behavior to variables not linked to alcohol use is also discussed to some extent. An examination of the influence of factors not linked to alcohol use will facilitate an assessment of the role of alcohol in violent encounters in relation to such factors. It is hoped that in this way a more balanced picture of the contexts and causes of violent behavior will emerge.

Perhaps a good strategy in attempting to clarify the reasons for the methods used in this study is (1) to point out some shortcomings or gaps in the methods of earlier studies on the connection between alcohol use and aggression; (2) to look at what an "ideal" study using survey methodology might look like; and (3) to explain my reasons for making compromises and deviating from this ideal, in order to move toward something approaching the optimal (given the practical restrictions inherent in the methods available and the subject matter at hand). Because of the subject matter, some attention is also given to methodological considerations and to the possibilities of bias in the data.

AIMS AND METHODS OF THE STUDY

The interview survey to be reported on was one part of a comprehensive multimethod study, as noted above. The total study utilized three different (and in several respects complementary) means of collecting data: (1) interviews with a representative sample of community residents; (2) a census of all incoming police reports during a 12-month period; and (3) systematic observations in 28 taverns and bars in the community. In order to clarify some aspects of the interviews, it is necessary to take a brief look at the design of the total multimethod study.

The specific methods and the types of samples selected for this study were decided on after weighing the following needs:

1. To arrive at estimates of the statistical involvement of alcohol use in different types of aggression events.
2. To get as complete a picture as possible of the factors affecting the relationship between alcohol use and aggression.
3. To check for biases inherent in the methods applied, and to maximize the validity of interpretations.
4. To include sufficient room for variation on central independent variables that may affect the relationship between alcohol use and aggressive behavior, especially sociocultural factors.
5. To study the interactional processes and situational characteristics that lead to inception, escalation, and de-escalation in aggressive incidents under the influence of alcohol.
6. To assist in the development of a research strategy in a widely scattered field.
7. To design the study in a way that would permit replication under different sociocultural and structural conditions.

A sampling universe that would have been ideal for theoretical purposes (and also some less ambitious explanatory objectives) would have been, of course, highly utopian. The reasoning below is only meant to provide a background to decisions that were bounded by methodological shortcomings, which themselves in turn are grounded in rather inflexible empirical (and ethical) strictures. Against the backdrop of the ideal, readers may also better appreciate the types of limitations to be taken into account in generalizing from the findings of this study and similar studies.

An ideal study designed to meet the objectives listed above would have had the following as sampling universes: (1) the set of *all* interpersonal acts of aggression, including acts of physical violence as a subset; and (2) the set of *all* drinking occasions (or, alternatively, all events in which one or more individuals were "under the influence of alcohol" or had a blood alcohol concentration above a certain specified limit) during a specific time period (or, even better, during different time periods so that historical variations would be available for sampling and analysis), with all relevant values on central variables available for analyses. In addition to providing comparative information on alcohol consumption during "typical" occasions of alcohol use (to be compared with consumption prior to violence), data from drinking episodes would provide a useful complement to data from violence episodes, since they would be sampled along the independent variable of alcohol use. This would enable a study of risk factors in connection with different types of drinking, and would provide more powerful analytical material than that possible with retrospectively sampled aggression episodes, which essentially would only allow the use of concordance measures (e.g., the proportions of events in which both alcohol use and violence occurred). In this book, however, I have had to be content with trying to extend the analytical possibilities of episodes of physical violence sampled after the fact.

For rather obvious practical reasons, the present study had to be limited to a geographically bounded sample within a specific time period. This limited the sample of episodes and behavior, as well as the participants in these episodes. My own residence in Canada, and considerations of access to funding, were primarily what led to taking samples out of the partial universes of aggression events and drinking occasions for people living in Canada. Given these restraints, the temporally and geographically truncated ideal would now have been to take samples representative of such events occurring for these residents during a specific time period.

Unbiased objective documentation of violence episodes, which would provide listings for sampling purposes, did not and does not exist. To try to set up such documentation through observational or other means would involve insurmountable difficulties and costs, not to mention ethical problems. It would probably also be subject to the uncertainty principle of measuring human conduct: Recording these social phenomena would at least to some extent change the phenomena themselves. Independent documentation that would permit a simple random sample of aggressive incidents or drinking situations cannot be instituted even for all aggression episodes (much less for all aggressive acts) during a specific time period in a limited area (unless studies are limited to very specific settings at very specific time periods, such as interactions in the taverns of a community). Instead, researchers must rely on *informants* of one kind or another, such as possibly the police, assailants, victims, or witnesses, to supply data on events of aggression.

Although it would be possible to design such a methodology prospectively, with informants reporting on new events as they occur, it is again likely that this would influence the behavior to be studied. This prospective methodology would also have to include quite a large sample of informants, and the problems in getting an unbiased sample of informants sufficiently motivated to take part would be considerable. The prospective strategy has been used for studying frequent, fairly predictable, and morally neutral occurrences (e.g., household consumption behavior). Since the present study was to be dealing with rather infrequent, morally controversial, and mostly highly unpredictable occurrences, a retrospective sampling method (i.e., sampling of a universe of episodes that had already taken place) had to be accepted.

In all probability, the most suitable informants for the purposes of this study would be individuals who took part in the behaviors and interactions constituting the episodes. Neutral observers would not be able to provide information on some central variables (e.g., the perceptions of the participants, their motives, attitudes, fears, etc.); furthermore, a great proportion of the events of interest in this case (e.g., most incidents of domestic aggression) would not have had any neutral nonparticipating observers. These considerations led to a further narrowing down of the possible sampling units and the universes of episodes from which to draw samples.

There would be rather narrow empirical limits to how much even informants who took part in the events under study could validly report. Memory lapses might well lead to incomplete and potentially biased reporting. In consequence, the sampling units had to be limited with regard to time period. Less than perfect recall also meant that methods were required for assessing at least roughly the extent of bias on central variables in the samples of aggression and drinking events obtained. These checks would not have been as necessary, had it been established in previous research that the informant method yields relatively unbiased information on aggressive acts and drinking occasions. This is not the case. On the contrary, it is known from interviews and mailed surveys (and even from the diary method) that a great deal of alcohol use in many populations remains unreported, partly because of recall errors (e.g., Lemmens, Knibbe, & Tan, 1988; Mäkelä, 1971; Midanik, 1982; Pernanen, 1974; Poikolainen & Kärkkäinen, 1983).[1]

In addition to recall errors, some respondents or informants might try to hide socially less desirable behavior. Previous research has found that stigmatized or normatively proscribed behavior is especially suscep-

1. Alcohol use is not in a unique position in this respect. The same kinds of biases have been found for cigarette smoking, the use of medical drugs, physician visits, serious life events, and numerous different types of consumer behavior (Asimakopulos, 1965; Cannell, Marquis, & Laurent, 1977; Carsjö, 1985; Gadourek, 1963; Loftus & Marburger, 1983).

tible to biases in reporting (Marquis, Marquis, & Polich, 1986; Pernanen, 1974; Wilson, 1981). This undoubtedly applies to at least some types of drinking and aggressive behavior (i.e., to both the main independent and dependent variables in this study). (Social desirability influences pertaining to the present study are discussed in Appendix A. Most of the analyses of recall errors will be presented in a subsequent cross-national report. It can be said here, however, that failure to recall violent episodes does not seem to have had much of a biasing effect on type of physical violence reported; see Pernanen, 1985.)

The reasoning presented above is not intended as a faithful reconstruction of the actual sequence of thinking when the study was set up, but rather a construct that should provide readers with a necessary background against which to check biases likely to appear in the data and to assess possible measures to counteract these biases. It will also perhaps aid in determining the generalizability of the findings and interpretations presented in this book.

Many of the reasons presented above were considered when it was decided to study the relationship between alcohol and aggression *in a single community*. A further consideration was that many research questions asked were previously unexplored, and a community format would better suit the pilot aspects of the project.[2]

SELECTION OF THE STUDY COMMUNITY

Criteria for selecting the study community naturally had to be weighed against each other. Highest priority was given to the following criterion: For the purposes of cross-national analyses, the locale should include large enough populations of one or more ethnic groups for which comparison data exist and/or for which further data could be collected. This was done in order to ensure extensions of analyses along cultural, structural, and attitudinal dimensions. The Finnish ethnic group was selected on the basis of its special interest for researchers investigating the link between the use of alcohol and aggressive behavior (see, e.g., Aho, 1976; Sariola, 1956; Verkko, 1951; Virkkunen, 1974). Because of this, and because of some other considerations related to geographical practi-

2. It is of course desirable that the results of this study, both those reported in this book and those reported in other publications, be replicated also for less limited sampling populations. In this context, a community study can serve as an intensive pilot study by providing information about variables of causal importance, about the validity of central measures, and so on.

cality and availability of support during fieldwork, the city of Thunder Bay in the province of Ontario was chosen as the site of the study.

The city is located on the northwest shore of Lake Superior. It is the western terminus of the St. Lawrence—Great Lakes Seaway and the gateway to the Atlantic for grain exports from the Canadian prairies. It has the world's largest grain-handling facility. Even more important economically than grain handling and shipping are the wood-processing industries: There are four paper mills and two major lumber-processing plants in the city. It is also the center for the regional government of Thunder Bay district, serving communities in a 350-mile radius in this sparsely populated area. The closest relatively large community is Duluth, Minnesota, about 200 miles to the south. The distance to the closest large Canadian city, Winnipeg, Manitoba, is 450 miles. The climate is northerly, with an annual average of +2.4° C (+36.3° F), a January average of −15.2° C (+4.7° F), and a July average of +17.5° C (+63.5° F).

Historically Thunder Bay is actually two cities, Fort William and Port Arthur, with a distance of about 2 miles between the city cores. Amalgamation took place in 1970. In the year 1981, the city of Thunder Bay had a population of approximately 112,500 (Ministry of Supply and Services Canada, 1983). Over two-fifths of the residents (49,000) were of British descent, but the community also has sizeable Finnish, Ukrainian, and Italian ethnic groups of about 10,000 each (Statistics Canada, 1978a; Raivio, 1975). In addition, there are 7,000 residents of mainly French descent and about 5,000 each of Polish, German, and Scandinavian (non-Finnish) origin. At the time of the study, about 18% of the population was born outside Canada, approximately 12% had immigrated during the preceding 35 years, and 4% had immigrated during the past 15 years (Ministry of Supply and Services Canada, 1983).

Additional criteria supporting the choice of this city as the site of the study were the following:

- The city was large enough to allow an intensive study with fairly large samples of respondents and subjects of observation, but without creating too much public awareness of the study; this could have counteracted its objectives and interfered with the normal flow of interaction and prevailing constellations of beliefs and attitudes.
- The community was large enough to provide a sufficiently large base of data on violent crimes during a period of 12 months.
- The city was relatively isolated geographically from other population centers, and thus not subject to great external influences and external sources of violence (e.g., nonresidents visiting the community in large numbers).

SELECTION OF THE INTERVIEW SAMPLE

The lower age limit for inclusion in the survey was first set at 18 (i.e., residents were to be included who turned 18 during the year of the inception of fieldwork), but the listings of community residents available at the time of sampling were relatively incomplete for the age groups under 20. For that reason, 20 was set as the lower age limit. There was no upper age limit, since it was felt important to get information on the experiences of violence among the elderly, probably the most vulnerable residents of the community. The selection of the sample, contacting of respondents, training of interviewers, and so forth have been described elsewhere in some detail (Pernanen & Carsjö, 1981).

A greater proportion of men than women were assumed to have been involved in aggression, and the response rate was expected to be lower for men. Consequently, an overselection of men over women was instituted. The original sample was designed to include 40% women and 60% men. Weighting procedures were planned to make the sample obtained representative of the city population as to gender distribution.

The sampling frame was the listing of residents and dwellings in the Henderson City Directory for the year preceding the inception of the study. In addition to the use of names listed in the directory, a complementary listing was based on the list of vacant dwellings in the directory. Additional names and addresses of residents were obtained by sampling these addresses and visiting them for enumeration purposes. Random substitutions were made at the time of interviewer contact in all cases if the selected persons or households had moved.

Since a response rate of 80% was set as a seemingly realistic goal, approximately 1,500 residents were to be selected as prospective respondents. A total final sample size of 1,200 residents of the city was determined for the survey. Out of these, 1,000 were to form a probability sample of Thunder Bay residents. The remaining 200 interviews were to be carried out with a specially selected sample of community residents of Finnish origin as part of the cross-cultural design of the study.[3]

In all, 1,479 persons were selected for the sample. Out of this total, 1,110 persons were interviewed. There were 187 random substitutions at the selected addresses because the selected persons in those cases had moved. These substitutions comprised 12.6% of the total selected sam-

3. A partly overlapping sample of 256 community residents of Finnish descent was obtained in this way. Very few of the findings of the analyses of this comparison sample are reported in this book. These findings will be reported separately in connection with results from the replication that is currently under way in a Swedish community.

ple. Out of the 1,110 completed interviews, 135 or 12.2% were conducted with substituted respondents. (No biases were found on central survey variables, such as experiences of violence and drinking patterns, as a result of this substitution procedure.)

In the representative sample of community residents (i.e., excluding the oversampled residents of Finnish origin), which constitutes the almost exclusive focus of this book, the selected sample consisted of 1,252 individuals. The final representative sample of community residents available for the present analyses consisted of 933 respondents. This indicates a response rate of 74.5%. Weighting for the undersampling of women gives us a weighted sample size of 979, which has been used in the presentation of data. The unweighted data have been used for the calculation of the statistical significance of estimates. For the interested reader, a discussion of reasons for attrition, an assessment of the representativeness of the final community sample, a presentation of the interview situation, and a discussion of several methodological validity checks are all available in Appendix A.

VIOLENCE THAT BECAME KNOWN TO THE COMMUNITY POLICE

Partly overlapping in time with the fieldwork of the interview survey (and the observational study) were the collection and coding of information by the Thunder Bay city police on all crimes of violence that came to their attention during a 12-month period (April 1, 1977–March 31, 1978) and were reported on "occurrence reports." The periods covered by police reports and by the retrospective interview data have different degrees of overlap, depending on the dates of interviews. Measured in calendar months, this ranges between approximately 0.5 and 6.5 months out of 12. Taking into account the actual distribution of interviews, the overlap, which ideally should be 100%, is in fact approximately 20%.

This lack of congruent coverage has not in all probability had much of a biasing effect on the results, since the rates of violent crimes did not differ very much over the two calendar years overlapping with the study period. The rate per 100,000 population was 1,013 in 1976 and 951 in 1977, which were the years in which varying 12-month periods were retrospectively covered in the interviews. In Table 3.1, the development of the rate of violent crime in the city over the period between 1976 and 1985 is shown (Statistics Canada, 1978b, 1979, 1980, 1981, 1982, 1983, 1984, 1985, 1986, 1987). In 1984 the Thunder Bay rate was the fourth highest among 11 Canadian cities with populations between 100,000 and 250,000. These had a mean violent crime rate of 887 per 100,000

TABLE 3.1. Rates of Violent Crime in the Study Community per 100,000 Population during the Years 1976–1985

Year	Rate per 100,000
1976	1,013
1977	951
1978	932
1979	811
1980	853
1981	967
1982	896
1983	1,059
1984	1,089
1985	1,074

population in that year. The rank had alternated between third and fourth during the preceding 8 years.

There are other imperfections of varying seriousness for comparisons between rates available from the interview study and the police record data:

1. For obvious reasons, no victimizations in homicides could be included in the events covered by the interview study sample. There were only two homicides in the police record sample of violent crime occurrences, however, and their impact on the results of comparative analyses is consequently minimal.

2. In the police record sample, an unknown number of robbery events, and some events in the categories of "other sexual offenses" and "other assaults," include incidents where actual physical violence did not occur. In some robberies a threat of violence, often connected with the showing of a weapon, sufficed for classifying the act as a violent crime. According to the Criminal Code of Canada, an event can be legally classified as a criminal assault if "he [a person] attempts or threatens, by an act or gesture, to apply force to the person of the other, if he has or causes the other to believe upon reasonable grounds that he has present ability to effect his purposes" (Zuber, 1974, p. 27). All in all, the total effect of these discrepancies also seems rather small, considering that there were only 57 cases of robbery and 16 cases of "other sexual assaults" among the census of 847 violent crimes. This means that from these two crime categories, an absolute maximum of 73 or 8.7% of the incidents could have been such that they contained no actual physical contact. (Most of the nonphysical crimes of violence would fit in under "threats" in the operational definitions of these episodes.)

3. A sampling discrepancy with greater potential impact was introduced by the fact that the incidents coming to the attention of the police included offenders and victims who were younger than the lower age limits in the interview study. Twelve years of age was defined as the lower age limit of the assailants in the violence episodes included in the interview study data. In nine cases, or 1.2%, of the violent crimes that came to the attention of the police (and for which the age of the offenders was known), the offenders were under the age of 12. Thus, this circumstance has had only a marginal effect on the results. These cases have been left out of analyses where appropriate.

The lower age limit of the respondents/victims in the questions pertaining to the preceding 12 months in the interview study was 18, since the youngest respondents interviewed turned 20 during the first year of the survey (and the reference period stretched back 12 months from the date of the interview). However, since the interviews were carried out late in the year, the lower age limit was 19 in the majority of cases. In comparing police record information with data from the 12-month reference period in the survey, I have excluded victims under the age of 19.

4. Some of the events in which the persons interviewed had been subjected to violence during the 12-month reference period had occurred outside the study community. By jurisdictional definition, this was not the case in any of the violent crimes that were reported to the police. There were no data that would allow a direct estimate of the proportion of victimization incidents reported for the 12-month period that occurred outside city limits. However, some estimates can be made from the subsample of respondents' most recent violent incidents that occurred during the 1-year period. These made up 43% of all the victimizations reported by the respondents for the 1-year period. Of these violence episodes, 94% had occurred in the community.

5. In all probability, a number of violent crimes taking place in the community involved individuals who resided outside its boundaries. Since the city is an economic and administrative center for a rather scattered population in the large surrounding area, it is perhaps not safe to conclude that city residents committed an equal number of violent crimes in other communities or jurisdictions, and that there would thus be a form of self-correction in the data. Unfortunately, the police record data did not include the places of residence for victims and offenders. Since the population in the surrounding area is small relative to the city population, this factor has probably not had a significant influence on the findings.

The breakdown of the 843 officially recorded aggression episodes as they appeared when sifted through the legal categories used by the police were as follows: homicides, 2 (0.2% of the total); woundings, 14 (1.7%);

assaults causing bodily harm, 197 (23.4%); other assaults, 549 (65.1%); rapes, 8 (0.9%); other sexual offenses, 16 (1.9%); and robberies, 57 (6.8%). When victims under age 19 and offenders under age 12 were omitted, in order to make the age criteria for sample selection equivalent to those for the violent incidents during the 1-year period covered in the interview sample, this left 781 occurrences of violent crimes in the community for later analyses.

With these precautions and caveats, I proceed in the next chapter to make some comparisons and joint analyses between the two sets of data covering the same approximate 12-month period. Some comparisons of a more problematic nature are made in later chapters between the *most recent* experiences of aggression of the city's residents and violent crimes that occurred during the 1-year period. Despite their difficulties, these comparisons still bring out interesting features of violence in the community.

4

The Prevalence of Violence and Threats of Violence

As a background to the later analyses of distinct episodes of violence, some generalizable data on the prevalence and incidence of aggression in the community are presented in this chapter. Such data were sought for two types of victimizations: (1) the number of times that a respondent had been the victim of physically violent acts during the 12 months immediately preceding the interview; and (2) the number of times during the same 12-month period that he/she had been subjected to threats of violence without violence ensuing in the same interactional episode. Partly for descriptive and cross-cultural purposes, and partly for methodological reasons, some questions were also asked about the witnessing of violence during the same 12-month period. Although episodes in which only threats of violence were made without any violence occurring are not discussed in later chapters of this book, the information on 12-month prevalence is of interest for the discussion of violent behavior in the community, and threats of physical violence thus receive parallel attention in this chapter. Acts of violence that were generally more serious than the ones covered in the interview survey are also looked at briefly in this chapter, through an analysis of data from the 12-month police census of violent crimes. A joint analysis of the information from police records and the interviews provides estimates on the "dark figure" (i.e., the proportion not officially reported) of violence as defined to the respondents. Such estimates are also made for male and female victims separately and for rough age groupings.

DEFINITIONS AND INTERVIEW PROCEDURES

Physical violence was defined operationally in the interviews by showing a listing of violent acts on a flash card and asking the interviewee to indicate on how many occasions he/she had been subjected to any of these acts (alone or in combination with other acts) during the 12 months preceding the interview. (See questions 3 and 4 in Appendix B for the list of violent acts presented to the respondent and the wording of questions asked.) The respondent was asked to disregard physical violence that was part of sports and games, or violence in the nature of "horseplay." It was made clear to the respondent that for the physical contact to be counted as violence, the assailant must clearly have shown the intention to hurt, or shown that he/she gave higher priority to reaching some other instrumental goal than to avoid hurting the respondent (e.g., as in pushing to get ahead in a line or in a purse-snatching incident). The throwing of objects was included as physical violence even if the respondent had not actually been hit by the object, as long as the antagonist had clearly shown that there was an intention to hurt the respondent physically.

Questions about incidents of mere threats of violence were also asked by using a flash card containing a list of specific types of threats (see questions 27, 28, and 29 in Appendix B). They were mainly included in the survey so that analyses could be carried out on aspects of aggression situations that increased or decreased the likelihood of escalation from threats into actual physical violence. The focus of this interest is on the role that alcohol use by the threatener and/or by the target of threats may play in this escalatory process. As in the questioning regarding actual violent acts, it was made clear in the instructions provided by the interviewer that threats made in a joking or half-serious mode were not to be included. In a parallel fashion to the definition of physical violence, threats were only counted if the respondent felt that there was a clear intention on the part of the antagonist to do physical harm to the respondent.

For witnessing of violence, the same categories of violent acts as for the personal victimization episodes were defined to the respondent by means of a flash card (see questions 55 and 56 in Appendix B). The same restrictive criteria as for personal victimizations were placed on the reporting of violence that was observed in real life (but not physically experienced) during the 12 months preceding the interview. Interviewees were asked not to include any violence that was part of sports or games, or that was in the nature of "horseplay;" in addition, no violence was included in which all participants were (or were judged to be) under the age of 15.

About a third of the adult population in the community had witnessed some form of violence during the 12 months immediately preceding the interview. As expected, only a small proportion of the population had themselves been subjected to violent acts during this period. The proportion of adult community residents who reported having been threatened with some act of physical violence without any violence resulting was even smaller.

GENDER IN RELATION TO ENCOUNTERS WITH AGGRESSION

Proportions of Men and Women Having Violence-Related Experiences

Considering what is now known about the prevalence of domestic violence and wife battering, it is not too surprising that there was no difference in the proportions of men and women who had been subjected to actual violence during the 1-year period. However, there were significant differences in the proportions of women and men who had been threatened with violence without any violence actually being committed. There were also substantial gender[1] differences in the likelihood of having witnessed physical violence. The findings on proportions of men and women who had experienced these forms of aggression are shown in Table 4.1. (The proportion of women victimized by violence is about the same as that subjected to physical abuse by spouses during any given year according to some U.S. studies [e.g., see Straus, 1986b].)

Information was obtained separately for two different types of threats: (1) threats with a weapon or object, and (2) verbal threats of hurting or killing the respondent. It was found that 3.0% of community residents had been subjected to the former kind of threat, while 6.9% had encountered verbal threats during the year preceding the interview. Overlap in one direction between these types of threat episodes was

1. I prefer to speak of "gender" instead of "sex," in part because the latter word has other connotations, but much more because I wish to emphasize the social and symbolic dimensions that are effective in determining differential attitudes and actions toward the genders/sexes, as well as the attitudes and the behavior of men and women themselves. Such differences no doubt to some extent have a biological grounding, but are greatly influenced by sociocultural factors, as a rich anthropological literature attests. In fact, the label "gender" as used in this book refers conjunctively to both the sociocultural and the biological aspects. Another linguistic problem related to gender is the use of "he" and "she," "his" and "her," and so forth. In contexts where the use of double pronouns would be too awkward or repetitious, only "he" is used from this point onward, especially when the gender distribution is such that males constitute a clear majority in the social or behavioral category discussed.

notable: A person threatened by the showing of a weapon had usually also been subjected to verbal threats of killing, maiming or hurting. Stated in absolute numbers, this means that 16 of the 25 persons in the sample who had been threatened with a weapon or object had also been threatened verbally. The extent to which this happened in the same situation is unknown.

A smaller proportion of women than men had been subjected to "empty" threats of physical violence (see Table 4.1). However, the women who had been subjected to threats were more likely than men to have been victimized in this way more than once during the year. Selecting out for special analysis only those individuals who had been threatened during the year provides a better view of this tendency; Table 4.2 shows this breakdown. A chi-square test showed that the distributions differed at the .05 level of significance ($\chi^2 = 6.30$, $df = 2$). A small proportion of women in the community were thus repeatedly subjected to serious threats that for one reason or another did not lead to violence in the same situation, possibly because many such threats were of a conditional nature ("If you don't . . . , I'll . . .") and the threatened women gave in to the demands or managed to neutralize the threats by other means. It should be pointed out that this pattern of concentration, although noticeable, was not at all as pronounced with regard to actual physical violence.

The mean number of violent incidents seen by the one-third of community residents who had witnessed any violence was 4.9. (The highest reported value in the range was an estimate of 55 such incidents.) Close to 10% of male witnesses and about 8% of female witnesses had seen 5 or more incidents of serious physical violence during the year; 5% and 3%, respectively, had seen 10 or more such episodes. It is to be expected that men, who more often work and move about outside the home, will have a higher likelihood of meeting, observing, and interacting with a greater number of people outside the home, and thus a higher probability of witnessing violent encounters (see Table 4.1).

TABLE 4.1. Proportions of Men and Women Who Had Experienced Different Forms of Aggression during a 1-Year Period

Form of aggression experienced	Men ($n = 495$)	Women ($n = 450$)	Total ($n = 945$)
Victim of violence	9.5%	9.2%	9.3%
Victim of threats	9.4%	5.6%	7.5%
Witnessed violence	38.9%	27.8%	33.6%
Any of these	43.2%	32.9%	38.2%

TABLE 4.2. Number of Episodes of Threats Experienced by Men and Women Who Had Been Threatened at Least Once during a 1-Year Period

Number of episodes	Men ($n = 41$)	Women ($n = 26$)	Total ($n = 67$)
One	51%	23%	40%
Two	27%	31%	29%
Three or more	22%	46%	31%

Male and Female Rates of Victimization

On the basis of the information given by the respondents about the number of occasions on which they had encountered aggression during the 1-year period, per capita estimates could be calculated for these experiences. The figures are a direct reflection of the overall *risk* of having these experiences for community residents aged 20 and over (Table 4.3). We have seen earlier that the proportions of women and men who were victims of one or more violent acts during a 1-year period were about equal; Table 4.3 shows that men and women also experienced the same mean number of actual victimizations (219 vs. 223 episodes per 1,000 women vs. men, respectively). In the Canadian Urban Victimization Survey, carried out in 1982 in seven major cities across the country, the rate of victimization for all violent incidents was 70 per 1,000 population aged 16 and over (i.e., only about a third of the rate of the present survey; Solicitor General, Canada, 1983). Women in the seven-city survey had an annual rate of 53 victimizations, and men had a rate of 90 victimizations, per 1,000 inhabitants. A major part of the difference is no doubt explainable by the lower threshold set for inclusion of violence episodes in the present study. However, the fact that the 1982 survey was carried out by telephone may explain some of the difference. Local idiosyncracies no doubt also have an influence on the discrepancy between these two sets of findings.

It is evident from Table 4.1 that a higher proportion of men than women had been subjected to mere threats during the 12-month period. With regard to *rates* of these incidents, a reverse pattern emerged: Women encountered almost twice as many incidents of empty threats as men (Table 4.3). This finding was foreshadowed earlier in a concentration of numerous threat episodes among relatively few women. The results regarding rates for the witnessing of violence follow the earlier-described pattern. Somewhat misleadingly, considering the large proportion of men and women who had not seen any violent incidents, it can be stated that men in the community had seen a mean of about 2 violent incidents during one year, while women had seen 1.2 such incidents.

TABLE 4.3. Number of Different Episodes of Aggression Experienced by Men and Women during 1 Year (per 1,000 Individuals Aged 20 and Over)

Form of aggression experienced	Men (n = 501)	Women (n = 452)	Total (n = 953)
Victim of violence	223	219	221
Victim of threats	241	440	340
Witnessed violence	2,022	1,234	1,646
Any of these	2,486	1,893	2,207

The much higher frequency of empty threats of violence directed against women is perhaps an indication of the use of such threats as a means of coercion by a man toward a woman in an intimate relationship, often in married life. In addition to its use in a conditional form in coercion, threatening may be part of structured (and even ritualized) conflict resolution. The fact that there is a greater difference between the risk of violence and the risk of threats among women may be explained by the fact that coercion by threats of violence is more "successful" when directed against women. Threatening a man may lead to actual physical violence in a greater proportion of incidents; this is reflected in the smaller discrepancy between the rates for violence and mere threats among men. To a much larger extent than is the case for a woman, a man's status and identity rest in physical prowess and ostensible fearlessness. He is expected to stand up to a threat.

AGE IN RELATION TO ENCOUNTERS WITH AGGRESSION

Proportions of Different Age Groups Having Violence-Related Experiences

Age was more strongly related to the risk of encountering violence and aggression than was a respondent's gender. The 12-month prevalence figures for the three types of aggression episodes all showed a decrease with increasing age (Table 4.4). A distinct drop in victimization by violence occurred at about age 40, and an equally clear drop occurred at about age 30 for mere threats. Witnessing of violence showed its greatest decrease at about the age of 30 and a rather even decrease in the older age groups. Over 60% of community residents in their 20s had either witnessed physical violence or been subjected to violence or threats during the year. As one might expect, youth was comparatively rich in aggressive experiences.

TABLE 4.4. Proportions of Individuals in Different Age Groups Who Had Experienced Aggression in Different Forms during a 1-Year Period

Form of aggression experienced	20–29 ($n = 233$)	30–39 ($n = 200$)	40–49 ($n = 156$)	50–59 ($n = 194$)	60+ ($n = 152$)	Total ($n = 935$)
Victim of violence	19%	12%	4%	4%	4%	9%
Victim of threats	16%	6%	5%	5%	3%	8%
Witnessed violence	58%	36%	30%	22%	11%	34%
Any of these	63%	42%	32%	25%	16%	38%

Among both men and women, individuals in their 20s had the highest rates of having been subjected to physically violent acts during the 1-year period: 21% among men and 18% among women. I have noted above that overall rates seemed to drop off after the age of 40 to a comparatively low level. There were indications that this drop occurred earlier among men than among women. In fact, the proportion of women in their 30s who had been victimized by physical violence was about twice that of men in the same age group (15% vs. 8%; not statistically significant). After the age of 40, men were about twice as likely as women to have been victimized by violent acts. The youngest adult men and women in the community had also been subjected to threats more often than any other age–gender group. The dominant finding related to these experiences of aggression is the comparatively high involvement of individuals under age 30, and especially males, as observers and participants in events of physical violence and as targets of threats.

The youngest residents of the city, in addition to having the highest prevalence rate of victimizations in violent encounters during the preceding 12 months, also had the highest rate of relatively frequent victimization. People in their 30s had intermediate rates, and the oldest residents had the lowest rates.

If we can assume that the probability of witnessing physical violence is an indicator of risk of personal involvement in serious aggression (or at least aggression outside the home), then it becomes apparent from Table 4.5 that the youngest respondents were more frequently present in settings involving relatively high overall risks of threats and violence. Of the youngest respondents, 16% had seen interpersonal violence five or more times during the year. Apparently, a subsegment of women in their 20s, 30s, and 40s were as likely to have seen five or more occasions of violence as men in the same age groups. The proportions were remarkably similar for men and women in these age groups.

TABLE 4.5. Proportions of Men and Women in Different Age Groups Who Had Witnessed Five or More Incidents or Physical Violence during a 1-Year Period

	20–29	30–39	40–49	50–59	60+	Total
Men	16% (123)	10% (113)	8% (92)	8% (93)	3% (80)	9.4% (501)
Women	15% (117)	10% (91)	8% (66)	3% (101)	0% (75)	7.6% (450)
Total	16% (240)	10% (204)	8% (158)	5% (194)	1% (155)	8.5% (951)

Note. n's for each group are in parentheses.

Women in their 50s and over, however, were considerably less likely than men of the same age to have witnessed violence frequently during the year.

Rates of Victimization in Different Age Groups

In discussing the relationship of risk of violence to age, I have thus far only used proportions of individuals who had encountered these experiences. For many purposes, however, it is preferable to count the total number of incidents encountered and to calculate estimates of central tendency. Since the ranges and standard deviations of these frequencies are relatively large, only two wide age categories have been used in the following analyses.

In Table 4.6, we see that individuals in their 20s and 30s were subjected to physical violence at a rate of 345 incidents per 1,000 residents per year. Younger women had the highest victimization risks of all for both threats (613 per 1,000) and actual violence (406 per 1,000). This means that the concentration of high rates of victimizations found generally among these women was particularly strong among young women. The victimization rate in violence for younger women was more than sixfold that of older women, while the threat rate was only twofold. Being subjected to threats without physical victimization thus decreased at a slower rate than did actual physical violence with increasing age among women. There was much more of a shift from the perpetration of physical violence to the making of mere threats against women than against men with increasing age.

In both age groups, women on the average were threatened with violence (without actual violence being committed) about twice as often as men. Both younger and older males witnessed more incidents of

TABLE 4.6. Number of Different Episodes of Aggression Experienced by Men and Women in Different Age Groups during a 1-Year (per 1,000 Individuals)

Form of aggression experienced	Men		Women		Total	
	20–39 ($n = 239$)	40+ ($n = 269$)	20–39 ($n = 214$)	40+ ($n = 250$)	20–39 ($n = 453$)	40+ ($n = 519$)
Victim of violence	291	162	406	62	345	114
Victim of threats	322	179	613	301	449	241
Witnessed violence	2,509	1,589	1,795	751	2,172	1,186
Any of these	3,122	1,930	2,814	1,114	2,966	1,541

physical violence than did women in corresponding groups. Young men in the community witnessed a mean of 2.5 incidents of violence during 1 year.

In the 1982 Canadian Urban Victimization Survey, the difference in victimization rates in violence between those under 40 and those over this age limit was even more pronounced; the rate was about sixfold in the younger age category (Solicitor General, Canada, 1985b), as compared to threefold in the present data. Here again, the difference in the criteria for defining violence, the discrepant methods of interviewing (telephone vs. personal interviews), and local variations probably explain the major part of the difference. The much higher risk of victimizations among the young is a global phenomenon, and is reflected in police and court records and in victimization studies based on surveys of general populations in numerous countries.

With rates available for both unfulfilled threats and actual physical violence it is possible to construct an aggregate measure of the gravity of threats encountered. Let V stand for the rate of actual incidents of violence experienced by a subgroup and T signify the rate of subjections to threats that did not lead to actual violence in the same period of time. The "gravity index" is given by the expression $V/V + T$. For present purposes, this ratio can be interpreted as an indicator of the tendency for threats to lead to actual violence; the higher the ratio, the higher the probability of physical violence once a threat had been made. One assumption underlying this interpretation is that there were no differences in the proportion of incidents of physical violence that were preceded by threats between the subgroups compared; that is, that the ratio between the number of violence episodes preceded by threats and the number of all violence episodes is constant for all subgroups. On the basis of this assumption, we can regard the ratio $V/V + T$ as an indicator of the seriousness of threats and/or the occurrence of interactional processes that facilitated the escalation of threat events into physical violence.

The greater the frequency of violence compared to the frequency of empty or nonconsequential threats, the greater this "gravity index" of threats should be. The maximum value would be unity (1.0) if all threats of violence were to lead to actual physical aggression, and the minimum value would be zero. Conversely, the nature of the measure can be characterized by the fact that the lower its value, the higher the proportion of "idle threats" in the group studied. Calculating from the data presented in Table 4.6 above produces the values shown in Table 4.7.

Apparently, the gravity of a threat in this sample was greater when directed against men than when directed against women. Furthermore, the seriousness of threats did not change with increasing age among men (at least not in the rough age groupings of Table 4.7), but showed a clear decrease among women. In other words, women over the age of 40 were much less likely to be subjected to physical violence when threatened with such than were younger women (and men, regardless of age). This finding may be explained by a greater relative prevalence of aggressive domestic incidents among older women. In any stable relationship, patterns develop for (among other things) conflict resolution, and compromises of individual objectives emerge that have to be negotiated over time. Interactional patterns (and especially aggression patterns) with relatively small variations have to be established, so that the stability of the relationship and of negotiated statuses and identities will not be overly threatened in each conflict situation. Such economy of conflict resolution (and other behaviors) relevant to the survival of the species is very prevalent among nonhumans (e.g., Bjerke, 1986; Lorenz, 1966).

Even in short-term relationships and in chance encounters humans usually prefer to avoid violence. This is all the more so in stable relationships, since the preservation of the relationship is at stake (unless violence also becomes institutionalized as part of a mutual adjustment pattern with its own functional role, as can happen in some extreme cases). Older women are more likely to have lived in these stable relationships for longer periods of time than are younger women, and

TABLE 4.7. "Gravity Index" of Threats Directed at Younger and Older Men and Women in the Community

	20–39	40+	Total
Men	.48	.48	.48
Women	.40	.17	.33
Total	.43	.32	.39

the acceptance of patterned ways of resolving conflicts may be a higher priority. Thus, threats of violence, as one fairly common resolution, are more likely to be accepted by women in such relationships, and a "normalized" way of ending verbal arguments may be to accept threats as the terminal point of a conflict. This patterning may occur in any enduring relationship. Younger women, on the other hand, less often have the same stake in accepting this type of resolution as the closure point of an interaction sequence. They encounter threats comparatively often in situations outside the home. There, escalation into violence may be more likely, because of the lesser availability of patterning and lower incentives for it. This would explain the higher value for younger women on the gravity index in Table 4.7.

The possible adjustment of the male counterpart in avoiding disruptive violence in the conflict situations of stable relationships should not be discounted, either. He may be less inclined to try to carry out his threats for some of the same reasons, and may more readily make a "generous" interpretation of the fact that his urgent wishes have been on the whole complied with. Because of the acceptance of the woman, he may also feel that a threat of violence is a relatively nondisruptive and "acceptable" way to end a conflict.[2] In some cases this type of negotiated definition never develops, and it can of course break down completely in acute conflicts. The effects of alcohol and excessive drinking patterns in such failures of human transactional processes should be of both practical and theoretical concern.

GENDER AND AGE VARIATIONS IN THE "DARK FIGURE"

Based on the 12-month police census of violent crimes, the rates of actual violent victimizations that came to official attention were 8.0 per 1,000 women and 8.2 per 1,000 men aged 20 and over. In the top half of Table 4.8, the rates are shown further broken down by gender and age. The differences between men and women in both age groups were small; age, on the other hand, was highly predictive of victimization that came to the attention of the police. Adults under the age of 40 were more than twice as likely to have been victimized in violent crimes as persons aged 40 and over. The general pattern is in fact reminiscent of the one found in the 12-month estimates from the interview study

2. This discussion is not meant to imply that mere threats and verbal abuse cannot at times be even more painful and damaging to a person and a relationship than some forms of physical violence.

TABLE 4.8. Rates of Officially Reported Violent Victimizations over a 12-Month Period per 1,000 Male and Female Residents of Different Ages, and Ratios of These Rates to the Rates Obtained through Interviews (Shown in Table 4.6)

	19–39	40+	Total
	Rates of violent crime (police reports)		
Men	10.9	5.4	8.2
Women	11.8	4.3	8.0
Total	11.3	4.9	8.1
	Ratio of police reports to survey estimates		
Men	1:27	1:30	1:27
Women	1:35	1:14	1:28
Total	1:30	1:22	1:27

(Table 4.6). However, the considerable dip among the older women was not found in the police report material.

The comparison with Table 4.6 shows that these figures are considerably lower than the 12-month rates of subjection to physical violence obtained in the interviews with community residents. In order to show the size of the discrepancies, the ratios between the estimates from police records and those obtained in the interview study have been calculated (Table 4.8, bottom half). By the rather inclusive criteria of physical violence employed in this study, only 1 of every 28 violent incidents in the community (or somewhat fewer than 4%) came to the attention of the police, and was subsequently recorded in their occurrence reports. It should be noted that many of the unreported episodes included acts of a relatively harmless nature, at least if we go by the nature of the acts themselves and the consequences in the form of injuries and medical care (see Chapters 7 and 8 for relevant discussions). The total context of some of these physically innocuous acts may, of course, still have been very serious, with grave consequences for the psychological well-being of the respondent and/or for the relationship in which it occurred.

The detection rate of about 4% is low, compared to figures obtained in most victimization surveys of violent crime. This has to be seen in the context of the milder forms of violence included in the operational definitions of this study (with the aim of getting a wide variation of severity of acts for analytical purposes). In typical victimization (and self-report) studies, attempts are made to include violence that would be considered serious enough by the police to warrant an occurrence report, or would have a substantial chance of leading to a conviction if brought to court. However, there are instances of even lower detection rates in the literature. One of the lowest reported is a rate of 0.3% for fighting and assault in a nonrandom sample of youths in Utah between the ages of 15 and 17 (Erickson & Empey, 1963). Coverage rates by police for common assaults generally range between 10% and 30%. For aggravated assaults, coverage rates of up to 70% have been obtained. In the Canadian Urban Victimization Study of 1982, the coverage rate of police reports was found to be 34% for assaults, 45% for robberies, and 38% for sexual assaults (Solicitor General, Canada, 1984).

A 1978 victimization survey in Sweden of a representative sample of the general population between the ages of 16 and 74 arrived at a coverage rate of 20% by the police for episodes of violence. This estimate was based on information provided by the respondents on whether the incidents had been reported to the police (Central Bureau of Statistics, Sweden, 1981). A good illustration of the joint magnitude of definitional problems, the discretionary powers of the police in recording violent incidents that come to their attention, and some social desirability effects in answering survey questions is the finding that in this Swedish study even a coverage rate of 20% would have overestimated the officially recorded crimes by more than 2½ times. According to police statistics, there were about 53,000 reported crimes of violence in Sweden in the study year. A projection from the survey gave an estimate of 135,000 violent incidents that were (allegedly) reported to the police. This type of overreporting of the involvement of police probably exists in other victimization surveys, which do not check the aggregated figures of their interview data against actual police reports.

In Table 4.8, we can see a relative underrepresentation of violent events involving young adult victims in the violence that came to the attention of the police. On the other hand, proportionately accurate representation did not seem to depend on whether the victims were male or female. The only ratio estimate that stands out in the table is the one for victimizations of women in their 40s or older, who had about double the reporting rate of the other age × sex groupings. This, like any other regularity in human behavior, can no doubt be explained by a combination of factors. When subjected to violence, women in this age group may be generally subjected to more severe acts than the other age groups. They may also be more likely to report their victimizations to the police, especially in "problem marriages" in which police often have to intervene several times a year.

Connecting the present finding to the earlier one shown in Table 4.7 (which indicated that women in the older age group received disproportionately more "empty" threats than younger women), we could also speculate that *when* violence occurs in the relationships of older women, it is seen as more serious and therefore is more likely to be reported. Violence in such cases may be more of a breach of conflict rules—and thus may imply more in transactional terms (perhaps creating a more severe shock)—in this age group, which has become accustomed to milder forms of aggression as terminal points in conflict. A related speculation is that the gravity index of threats is low among older women precisely because threateners know that the probability of the police's being informed is relatively high. At this stage nothing definite can be said about the validity of these different types of explanations, but they seem to open up interesting and useful research questions.

OBSERVING VIOLENCE: LOCATIONS AND TYPES OF ACTS

Locations and Settings

A majority of residents, many of whom had not themselves seen any violence during the preceding 12 months, had definite opinions about where violence was to be found in the community. When asked to name areas or locations in the city "where there is more violence than [in] most other parts of the city" (see question 105 in Appendix B), a minority (30%) expressed a lack of knowledge in words such as "I don't know, I don't go out at night and I have no trouble"; "I have seen enough fighting in my own home—I don't go out at all"; or "I don't know of any since I hardly go into the city—just for shopping twice a week." Very few (4%) felt that there really were no specific areas where violence was more likely to occur: "It's the same all over"; "It's all the same pretty much—the variations in danger are pretty slight"; "All the streets at night"; "It's all over—there are gangs, old and young, hanging around pool rooms with nothing to do."

A substantial proportion (18%) named specific public drinking places in the city (25% of those who mentioned any type of area or location at all). There were also some vaguer references (8%) to "some hotels and drinking places," "every mixed bar in town," "closing time at any local bar," "bars and taverns with a young population," "cheaper bars," "grubby hotels," and the like.[3] Thus, 26% of community residents thought rather spontaneously of public drinking establishments as locations where a disproportionate share of violence in the community

3. A policeman offered a partly dissenting opinion: "Newer drinking places are sometimes worse. The violence that goes on in the dives is less sadistic, just clumsy."

occurred. If those who did not know of any such areas are omitted from the calculations, the proportion is 37%. In addition, another 32% named streets and areas with a great concentration of taverns and bars, especially those frequented by youths, the poorer segments of the working class, "skid row" groups, or native Indians. Even persons who disqualified themselves from expressing a definite opinion on specific areas or locations with a heightened risk of violence framed this in such terms as these: "I don't know of any areas, since I don't frequent drinking areas"; "I don't really know of areas here—I don't go to public places now"; or "I don't go to hotels except for banquets and I just don't know."

Exclusive references to areas that did not point as clearly to alcohol use in general and drinking in public places in particular were much fewer and included areal designations such as "the waterfront," by the railway tracks," "in the coal docks," "downtown areas with gangs," "areas with back lanes," "any dark secluded area in any place," "depressed areas, townhousing areas," "low-income housing areas," and so forth. More inclusive references also included "downtown," "city center," "the east end," and the like. A number of respondents expressed a lack of personal experience as a basis of their assessments and referred to the newspapers, "news," or hearsay as their main source of information.

Also, when community residents were asked about locations where they had seen violence during the last 12 months (question 57 in Appendix B), the most commonly mentioned locations were public drinking places. At least one episode of physical violence had been observed in such locations by 17% of the adult population (Table 4.9). I have noted earlier that about a third of the residents, (approximately

TABLE 4.9. Proportions of Men and Women Who Had Witnessed Violence in Various Locations during a 1-Year Period

Location	Men ($n = 507$)	Women ($n = 463$)	Total ($n = 970$)
Own home	3.6%	3.0%	3.3%
Other home	5.5%	7.3%	6.4%
Work or school	8.3%	3.9%	6.2%
Public drinking place	22.3%	11.9%	17.3%
Street or park	15.6%	13.0%	14.3%
Some other place[a]	4.7%	1.9%	3.4%

[a]This category includes sports arenas, restaurants not licensed to serve alcohol, summer cottages, bush camps, buses and cars, hotel rooms, stores and plazas, etc.

39% of men and 28% of women) reported having witnessed any interpersonal violence during the year. Thus about half (52%) of those who had witnessed any violence during the year had done so in public drinking places (often in addition to other locations).

More than 1 in every 5 men had seen violence in a public drinking place during the year; among women, slightly more than 1 in 10 had done so. These results pertain to the total sample of respondents, including those who were abstainers or otherwise did not visit drinking places. Among community residents who had drunk alcohol in a public drinking establishment at least once during the past year, 27% of men and 17% of women had seen tavern violence (23% of the total sample).

Although some of the violence observed by residents during the year probably took place outside the city, including some taverns and bars in other communities, most occurred in drinking places within the community itself. Some inferential data in the present study may help clarify the extent to which violent incidents in which city residents were involved took place outside city limits. These data pertain to the residents' most recent episodes of victimization by violence, which, as has been pointed out earlier, constitute a central focus of analysis in later chapters. Information on the geographic locations of the incidents was available for these. A total of 93 of these violence episodes had occurred within the preceding 12 months, and were thus covered by the question on violence during this period. Of these, 87, or 94%, took place in the home community. If we assume that these most recent episodes of violence are roughly representative of all the 214 victimizations that the respondents reported having experienced during the 1-year period, we can conclude that the vast majority of these victimizations occurred in homes, public drinking places, streets, parks, malls, parking areas, and so on, located within the city limits.

In reading Table 4.9, it should be kept in mind that the figures do not directly reflect the actual prevalence of violent events in the different locations, for two predominant reasons:

1. The probability of anybody's witnessing a violent incident is directly related to the *number of people present* in the location (and in a position to observe at least part of the violent encounter). Thus, there was a much higher chance for any violent event to be reported in the survey if it occurred in, for example, a tavern than if it occurred in a private home. In fact, the likelihood of two or more sampled community residents' reporting on the *same* event was much higher for violent incidents in taverns and streets or parks than for incidents in private home. Many occasions in a private home have no adult witnesses, while those in a public drinking place often have 30–40 or more witnesses, all of whom are potential informants on the same incident. To get at a

more accurate estimate of actual prevalence in different locations from data on witnessing such occurrences, we would have to inversely weight the results in Table 4.9 by the number of people in a position to make the observation.

2. The likelihood of observing any event in any location is also directly proportional to the *time spent* by potential witnesses in these settings. This weighs down the prevalence and incidence figures for locations such as streets, parks, and public drinking places, and works in favor of homes and workplaces, where people on the average spend a larger share of their waking hours.

The remarks above should alert us to the biases that arise from all estimates based on reported observations of events. They have their significance, however, if correctly interpreted. In addition to their use for comparative purposes, the importance of estimates of episodes witnessed resides in the fact that they probably reflect our conceptions about the true extent and nature of aggression, without any attempts at corrective weighting for biasing factors on our part. Thus, street violence may be given disproportionate emphasis as a social problem because of this natural overweighting in observations. The surprise expressed at the discovered universality of family violence is, of course, understandable in this light.

The findings of Table 4.9 can be seen as a partial test of the hypothesis that differential exposure (time at risk) determines the prevalence of witnessing violence by men and women. With regard to violence observed in public drinking places, the pattern seems to tally fairly well with such a modest common-sense hypothesis. Somewhat surprisingly, however, men did not have a lower rate of observing violence in their own homes. Beyond a threshold value, time spent in a location is thus not a major determinant of observing violence during a given time period. Instead, the nature of a location probably only determines the likelihood of socially visible violence in conjunction with the characteristics of the individuals present, types of activities and social interaction taking place, and the like. This fact comes out even more clearly when locations for observing violence are related to the ages of observers (see Table 4.10).

Almost two-thirds of those who had observed violence in the preceding 12 months had made such observations in only one type of place, and almost one-fourth in two types of places. Among the respondents who had witnessed acts of violence during the past year, one-quarter had seen it *only* in a public drinking place (29% of men and 18% of women). The second most common single place for witnessing violence was a street or park. It was the most frequent place for women to have observed violent acts (20% of those having witnessed violence,

TABLE 4.10. Proportions of Community Residents in Different Age Groups Who Had Observed Violence in Different Locations at Least Once during a 1-Year Period

Location	20–29 ($n = 243$)	30–39 ($n = 208$)	40–49 ($n = 160$)	50–59 ($n = 197$)	60+ ($n = 156$)	Total ($n = 964$)
Own home	3%	5%	3%	3%	1%	3%
Other home	13%	6%	5%	3%	2%	6%
Work or school	10%	6%	8%	3%	1%	6%
Public drinking place	40%	17%	9%	7%	3%	17%
Street or park	26%	15%	10%	10%	6%	14%
Some other place	7%	2%	2%	4%	1%	3%

compared to 17% of men). The three combinations of having witnessed violence in a public drinking place, a street/park, or both locations accounted altogether for more than half of the combinations of locations where violence had been observed. There was no difference between men and women in this proportion. The greatest gender difference was found among those who had witnessed violence only in somebody else's home, with 13% of women and 3% of men having done so exclusively. Out of the total sample (witnesses and nonwitnesses), about 13% of men and 10% of women had seen violence in two or more types of locations; 5% of men and 2% of women had witnessed violence in three or more kinds of places (out of the six categories listed on the flash card).

It has been noted earlier that a much larger proportion of the younger adult residents of the community had observed violence than had older residents. This could be explained by the fact that young people spend more time in locations where violence is more likely to occur, such as outside in streets and parks or in taverns and bars. The results show, however, that the youngest age group had the highest rates of witnessing violence in all locations except in their own homes, for which they equaled the mean prevalence rate for the total sample (Table 4.10). In almost all locations, there was a rather steady decrease with age in the percentage of individuals who had seen violence during the year. The high exposure to violent acts among young adults is therefore not a function of the time that they spend in any one type of location, but rather the company they keep (especially members of their own age group), the activities they participate in, their typical interactions within the group, and so forth. These factors are to some extent independent of the location in which they happen to be. Young adults probably also have slightly different rules regarding permissible settings than do older age groups, as well as a generally lower threshold for open conflict.

The percentages of individuals who observed violence in two or more locations showed age patterns consistent with those emerging from the earlier results. Thirty-one percent of the youngest men and 23% of the youngest women had seen violence in more than one type of location. In the age group with the next highest proportions, the 30- to 39-year-olds, about 12% of both men and women had done so, and only 1% of the residents aged 60 and over had.

Types of Violent Acts Observed

Respondents were asked about the types of violent acts that they had observed (see question 55 in Appendix B). This was again done by presenting them with a flash card that listed the different types of violent acts. Table 4.11 displays the proportions of city residents who had observed these different acts at least once during the year. The fact that a smaller proportion of women had seen an episode of violence confounds the assessment of gender-specific patterns in the acts seen. This has been taken into account in comparing the genders in the table. In this comparison, only people who had observed at least one type of violent act are included.

More men than women had seen all the different types of acts that were listed on the flash card (not including the open-ended category of "hurt somebody in some other way," referred to in Table 4.11 as "other violent acts"; a great variety of acts were included in this category: "Pulling hair," "Biting and scratching," "Pouring boiling coffee on an

TABLE 4.11. Proportions of Respondents and of Male and Female Witnesses Who Had Observed Different Types of Violent Acts at Least Once during a 1-Year Period

		Witnesses only		
Type of violent act	Respondents ($n = 972$)	Men ($n = 206$)	Women ($n = 134$)	Total ($n = 340$)
Hitting with weapon or object[a]	8.4%	28%	22%	26%
Punching/hitting with fist	24.7%	83%	62%	75%
Kicking	17.6%	54%	52%	53%
Throwing of object at somebody	6.9%	21%	22%	21%
Slapping	19.3%	55%	64%	58%
Grabbing, pushing, or shoving	20.6%	61%	64%	62%
Other violent acts	3.9%	12%	11%	12%
One or more types of violent acts	35.0%	100%	100%	100%

[a]Weapons and objects used included knives, two-by-fours, shoes, pop bottles, etc.

innocent bystander," "Two teenagers were trying to rob an old man," "While driving I saw a man jump on top of another man and hit him," "A glass was kicked in a fellow's face," and the all-inclusive statement "You name it"). The male predominance was highest for observations of hitting with a fist and hitting with a weapon or object (as measured by male–female ratios of the prevalence figures).

Generally, there was a slight tendency for women to have seen more of the types of acts that were used against women and by women (see Chapter 7), perhaps because women are more likely to participate in social settings where other women are present, and men in settings where there is a greater than average proportion of other men.

Acts observed by witnesses of different ages show no surprising patterns in the light of earlier findings. Of the youngest adults (ages 20–29), 81% had seen hitting with a fist, while 71% of witnesses in their 30s and 65% of witnesses aged 40 and over had. The same type of decrease with increasing age was evident for kicking (64%, 44%, and 41%, respectively). Except for throwing of an object at somebody (25%, 16%, and 17%, respectively), there was very little difference among witnesses from the three age groups in observing the other types of acts.

ALCOHOL USE PATTERNS AND EXPERIENCES OF AGGRESSION

If participation in alcohol use events within a society increases the likelihood of having encountered aggression as either a victim or a perpetrator, one would expect individuals who drink more often or drink more often in a certain manner (e.g., amounts above a threshold level) to have had more experiences of aggression during the preceding 12 months (Aromaa, 1977a). On a common-sense time-at-risk basis, it can also be predicted that frequent drinkers, especially individuals who frequently drink in premises licensed to serve alcohol, will have a higher likelihood of witnessing violence in such places. Whether a greater proportion of these people will also have observed violence in other places is a more interesting substantive question.

In the present study, there was no clear-cut relationship between the typical drinking frequency of the individual and the three types of experiences of aggression during the preceding year. The proportions of persons subjected to acts of violence during the year ranged from 13% for those who drank alcohol at least three times a week to 7% for the least frequent drinkers (those drinking at the most once a month). The differences were more pronounced with regard to observing violence, where individuals drinking once or twice a week showed the highest prevalence figure. A similar, but weaker, tendency existed for subjections to threats.

There was a high relative frequency of witnessing violence among those who drank once or twice a week. This may indicate a pattern of weekend drinking, perhaps predominantly in public settings, where the probability of seeing violent encounters is especially high. Analyses showed that this category of alcohol users also included a disproportionate number of young adults, and we have already seen that they are more likely both to be present as observers in episodes of aggression, and to participate actively themselves in such situations. The point that this discontinuous finding should make clear is that, even though a statistical connection between alcohol use and aggressive encounters seems very likely in many jurisdictions and cultural spheres, we should not expect a linear relationship between frequency of drinking and these experiences. Above all, we would have to take into account the differing distributions of episodes in which more than a certain amount of alcohol is consumed or consumption leads to a surpassed threshold blood alcohol concentration, where the risk of aggressive behavior may begin to increase. Even this does not suffice, however. We have to examine the differential distributions of settings and social contexts in which the drinking occurs. These of course differ from one country or region and subgroup of the population to another. In addition, we ought to take into account the differential "social meanings" that drinking generally has in a group of people, as well as how the more immediate effects of alcohol may interact with these and perhaps other definitions (which on the surface may seem unrelated to the business of having a few drinks in the neighborhood tavern, or a night out with the boys).

In the present study, men in the community drank considerably more often than women did. Such a gender-specific pattern in the frequency of alcohol consumption has been found in numerous surveys of drinking habits in many different parts of the world. Here it could explain the greater probability of observing violence and of being subjected to threats among the individuals who drank more often. A rather blunt cross-tabular test of whether the confounding causal role of gender could explain the relationship between a dichotomized drinking frequency (with the cutoff at drinking once per week) and encounters with violence and threats was carried out. The result was a partial specification of the relationships to one of the genders: For all three types of encounters with aggression during the year (subjection to acts of violence, subjection to threats, and the witnessing of violence), a greater proportion of the more frequent male drinkers had greater exposure than less frequent drinkers and abstainers. The difference was statistically significant for physical violence ($\chi^2 = 5.84$, $df = 1$, $p < .05$), but not for threats ($\chi^2 = 3.06$, $df = 1$, $p < .10$). Among women the relationship was less clear. With violence it was in fact reversed, but not at a statistically significant level. This no doubt can be explained at least in part by the domestic nature of female victimizations.

Among both men and women, the individuals who drank once or twice a week were more likely than even the most frequent drinkers (those drinking three or more times per week) to have observed violence during the preceding 12 months. Most conspicuous was the high proportion of persons in this drinking category who witnessed violence on 10 or more occasions during the year: 13% as compared to 4% of men and women who drank nearly daily or more often. These findings can probably be explained partly by the age distribution of individuals in the frequency of drinking categories. Low levels of witnessing violence among abstainers and very infrequent drinkers are inherent in the life style of these individuals, particularly since this group includes a disproportionate number of older people. Similarly, many individuals who consume alcohol every day or nearly so every day will do so mainly in their own homes, and (by tradition, cultural preference, or inertia) typically in connection with meals. The "weekend drinkers," on the other hand, who are included among those who drink two or three times per week, use alcohol disproportionately in connection with partying, visits to public drinking places, or other special weekend events.

These interpretations are corroborated in part by the fact that while about 30% of the twice-a-week drinkers had observed violence in drinking establishments, only 17% of more frequent drinkers had ($\chi^2 = 6.68$, $df = 1$, $p < .01$). Equally revealing is the fact that 22% of the former group had seen violence in streets and parks, while only 9% of the latter category had ($\chi^2 = 8.74$, $df = 1$, $p < .01$). The high rate of witnessing violence in a street or park also fits in with an active, youthful life style, when probably more time is spent out in the city than during other phases of the adult life cycle. An equally consistent and clear-cut result was the least frequent drinkers' low prevalence of observing violence in *all* locations.

The findings presented in the top half of Table 4.12 show that the frequency with which the respondent had visited a public drinking place during the 30 days preceding the interview (which probably at least ordinally reflects the pattern of consumption in taverns and bars over longer time periods in a sufficiently reliable way) was strongly related to the probability of witnessing violent incidents. Although the strongest relationship, as expected, was with witnessing violence in a public drinking place, there was a rather weak but broad tendency toward higher rates of observing violence in other places, including the home setting.

TABLE 4.12. Number of Occasions When Violence Was Observed, and Locations Where Violence Was Observed, by Community Residents During a 1-Year Period as Related to the Number of Days on Which They Had Visited a Public Drinking Place in the Last 30 Days (Nonabstainers Only)

	Visits to drinking place in the last 30 days						
	At no time	1 day	2 days	3–4 days	5–9 days	10–30 days	Total
	($n = 264$)	($n = 185$)	($n = 115$)	($n = 105$)	($n = 90$)	($n = 48$)	($n = 807$)
Number of times violence observed in past 12 months							
At least once	22%	32%	39%	45%	57%	63%	36%
3 or more times	8%	12%	11%	20%	25%	35%	14%
5 or more times	5%	9%	8%	11%	17%	19%	9%
10 or more times	3%	3%	3%	5%	10%	8%	5%
Location where violence seen at least once							
Own home	4%	4%	3%	2%	4%	6%	4%
Other home	6%	6%	8%	9%	10%	8%	7%
Work or school	6%	7%	5%	7%	11%	10%	7%
Public drinking place	7%	13%	16%	31%	41%	55%	19%
Street or park	12%	12%	19%	22%	22%	18%	16%
Some other place	2%	4%	5%	6%	6%	0%	4%

These results taken together indicate that frequency of alcohol use per se is not nearly as strongly related to the probability of being in settings and situations with high risk of violence as is the patterned cluster of these factors: alcohol use, specific location of use, and connected activities, participants, and expectations. The same type of pattern was also found in the 1982 Canadian Urban Victimization Survey, where the average number of evening activities outside the home was strongly related to risk of becoming a victim of violence (Solicitor General, Canada, 1985b). This finding held up even after a control for age (which was negatively correlated with out-of-home activities in the evening) was instituted.

DETERMINANT PATTERNS IN RECENT EXPERIENCES OF AGGRESSION

Logistic regression analyses were performed with the three different experiences of aggression during the past year as dependent variables. Logistic regression models are useful in analyzing the influence of a set of dichotomous variables—for example, the variable "whether alcohol was used by the assailant or not" (a) and "whether the assailant was male or not" (m)—on a dichotomous dependent variable, such as "whether the victim was injured in violence or not" (i). The logistic model specifies that the risk of injury depends on such a set of independent variables as follows: $p(i) = 1/\{1 + \exp(-[\beta_0 + \beta_1(a) + \beta_2(m)])\}$. On the basis of the beta coefficients and the presence or absence of a characteristic (e.g., assailant's being male or not being male, assailant's having consumed alcohol or not having consumed alcohol), it is possible to predict the relative risk (or "odds ratio") between sets of characteristics that the dependent variable will occur (in this case, the victim's being injured). We can, for example, answer this question: "How much does the risk of injury to the victim increase or decrease between violent episodes in which the assailant is a male who has been drinking, compared to when the assailant is a sober female?" In addition to such relative risk calculations, we can examine the relative importance of individual factors (in a set of factors) by noting the confidence level at which the beta coefficients differ from zero. In the logistic regression analyses reported in this book, the CATMODE procedure in the SAS statistical package was used (SAS Institute Inc., 1985). This procedure estimates the value of the beta coefficients by a maximum-likelihood method, and tests the goodness of fit of the model on the data with a chi-square test. A good introduction to the theory and application of the logistic model is provided by Schlesselman (1982).

Table 4.13 presents a composite picture of findings from several logistic regression models fitted on the data. The factors were ranked from 1 to 5, indicating the relative importance of the factors in determining the risk that an individual would be subjected to violent acts or mere threats of such in a 12-month period, and that he/she would observe violence during the same period. The rank order was calculated on the basis of the mean of the ranks in the models fitted on the data (only models employing at least four different main effect variables were included). The significance level was the modal one (i.e., the level achieved by the variable more often than any other level in the models fitted). The factors were introduced serially and showed great consistency between different models in their determinant strength and their level of significance. The numbers after the plus and minus signs in the table show the relative rank of the absolute value of the standardized beta coefficient for the factor in the respective models. A plus sign in front of the rank designation means that the factor (among the constellation of factors included in the models) had a risk-increasing effect, and a minus sign means that it tended to decrease the risk of these episodes' occurring.

Of the factors studied, being young had the strongest and most consistent influence on all three types of encounters with violence, increasing the risk more than any other factor. Married status was consistently in second place, decreasing these risks. Being male did not have any effect on the likelihood that a person would be subjected to some type of violent act or acts on at least one occasion during the year.

TABLE 4.13. Summary of Rank Order, Direction, and Statistical Significance of Risk Factors in Different Logistic Regression Models Determining Risk of Being Subjected to Violence and Threats and of Observing Violence at Least Once during a 1-Year Period

Risk factor	Witnessing violence	Subjection to threats	Subjection to violence
Male	+3***	+3	0
Aged under 30	+1****	+1****	+1****
Married	−2****	−2*	−2**
Education: at least finished grade 12	+4***	0	0
Drank alcohol at least three times/week	0	0	+3*
Drank alcohol once or twice per week	+5**	0	0

*$p < .05$.
**$p < .01$.
***$p < .001$.
****$p < .0001$.

On the other hand, it had a strong effect on the probability of observing violence, and a nearly significant influence on the risk of encountering mere threats of violence at least once during the year. Higher than average education increased the probability that a person would observe violence at a statistically highly significant level (and it did so independently of the effect of age). The influence of a "weekend drinking" pattern also increased the likelihood that violence would be witnessed, but the standardized beta coefficients were generally weaker than for all the background variables included in the logistic regression models. Drinking frequency was not associated with the risk of being subjected to threats of physical violence, whereas relatively high drinking frequency increased the risk of being physically assaulted (at the .05 level of significance).

Table 4.14 presents the beta coefficients of the logistic regression models that had the best fit on the data, and the statistical significance levels indicating the confidence with which it could be asserted that they differed from zero. The statistical significance of the goodness-of-fit test (displayed at the bottom of the table) is a reversal of the common type of indication, in that a high probability level indicates a good fit and a low one represents statistically unacceptable levels. Somewhat better fits were available for two-factor models, but for illustrative purposes at least three characteristics of participants are presented as independent factors in the models. The fit of the models was relatively good for experiences of violence and threats, and they have been included in the table. The best-fitting model predicting the witnessing of violence did not have a satisfactory fit, and no model is displayed for the accounting of this experience.

On the basis of the models of Table 4.14, some relative risk calculations can be made in order to illustrate predicted differences in risk between some population groups. Let us choose the extreme groups for comparison. With regard to subjections to threats, the extreme groups were the same as for witnessing violence, except that educational level did not have any predictive power. The model in Table 4.14 predicts that unmarried young males would have a 0.24 risk during a 1-year period of being threatened with physical violence without violence actually coming about. The corresponding risk for married women over the age of 30 would be 0.03. Thus the former segment of the population would have an eightfold risk of encountering such threat episodes. It should perhaps be pointed out that since we are dealing with proportions of the population and not rates of subjections to threats, the small group of women who were frequently subjected to threats does not influence the results in proportion to its numbers of victimizations.

TABLE 4.14. Determinants of Risks of Becoming a Victim of Threats and Physical Violence during 1 Year, According to Logistic Regression Models (Values of Beta Coefficients and Their Significance Levels)

	Subjection to threats		Subjection to violence	
Risk factor	β	p	β	p
Male	+0.62	.0179	[a]	
Aged under 30	+1.07	.0001	+1.03	.0001
Married	−0.63	.0195	−0.69	.0046
Education: at least finished grade 12	[a]		[a]	
Drank alcohol at least three times a week	[a,b]		+0.59	.0146
Drank alcohol once or twice a week	[a,b]		[b]	
Intercept	−2.85	.0001	−2.35	.0001
Likelihood ratio test for goodness of fit	$\chi^2 = 3.27$, $df = 4$, $p = .5137$		$\chi^2 = 4.39$, $df = 4$, $p = .3553$	

[a]Including this factor in the model led to a less satisfactory fit, and it was therefore excluded.
[b]Only one of the two drinking frequency variables was included in each separate logistic regression model.

The risk of being victimized in episodes of actual physical violence was not influenced by the gender of the person. Thus, the primary contrast is that between unmarried individuals under the age of 30 who drank alcohol at least three times a week and married individuals over 30 who drank less often than three times per week on the average. For the former group the risk would be 0.32 and for the latter group 0.05, yielding a more than sixfold relative risk. (Finally, in the case of observing violence, it should just be mentioned that the highest-risk category would be unmarried males under the age of 30 with a higher than median education who drank alcohol once or twice a week. Conversely, the lowest-risk group would be married women over the age of 30 with a lower than median education who were not "weekend drinkers.")

Based mainly on the findings summarized in Table 4.13, it can be said that drinking alcohol once or twice per week, which represents youthful weekend drinking to a disproportionate degree, is linked to presence in settings where visible violence occurs. More frequent drinking, however, is positively related to the risk of being subjected to violent acts.

5

Violence Episodes: Participants, Settings, and Relationships

This chapter examines characteristics of actual violence episodes available from the interviews and the records kept by the police. The data presented here are meant to serve as a background to the later analyses of the involvement of alcohol. The sampling procedure used in the interview survey as it applies to individual episodes is discussed first.

THE SAMPLING OF EPISODES IN THE INTERVIEW STUDY

In the interview survey, it was not possible to get episode-specific information for a direct probability sample of violent events that occurred within a delimited time period. One reason was the concentration of aggression episodes among relatively few individuals, and the consequent problems for these individuals in remembering and reporting (and for the interviewer in recording) details for each of the incidents during, say, the 12 months immediately preceding the interview. In a probability sample of episodes, the skewed distribution of violence in the population would also lead to narrow ranges of variation on several important variables that could contribute to the relationships between alcohol use and aggression. The resulting sample of actors would be self-weighting with regard to the probability of their being implicated in occurrences of violence (i.e., there would be a heavy overrepresentation of young males, individuals from "skid row" subcultures, members of "problem families," etc.). If the main aim of the study were to describe episodes of violence as they occurred in the community (and if the practical problems mentioned above could be overcome), the procedure would be ideal. However, because I wanted to carry out analyses that would provide theoretical insights regarding the role of situational, demographic, and other factors in determining the linkage between alcohol use and aggression and in molding the characteristics of alcohol-related aggression, I felt that the study would be better served by more variation on these variables. A greater number of cells in a quasi-factorial setup would be covered in this way. On the other hand, this makes the episode samples somewhat artificial and not redeemable by greater control over the variation in these "expanded" variables (as would be the case in experimental setups).

For the reasons mentioned, most data for the analyses of specific episodes of violence in the interview study were provided by samples of the *most recent* events in the experience of the respondents. There are powerful precedents for this sampling procedure. In experimental research in psychology and other disciplines, unweighted analysis of samples of "the most recent episode" is in effect accepted practice, since such studies are not concerned with representative description, but attempt to test substantive hypotheses with direct theoretical implications. In choosing subjects for experimental research and analyzing data from such research, no weighting procedures are instituted for generalizability purposes. Persons who drink alcohol once a week get the same weight with regard to their reactions in experiments that test the effect of alcohol on aggression as do persons who drink every day, and individuals who react aggressively in a disproportionate number of drinking events are also not "weighted up" with the aim of generalizing the results to real-life occurrences. In addition, despite the common limitation of the subject samples to "social drinkers," inferences are generally drawn that cover all drinkers and drinking situations (vaguely within the parameters specified by the experimental paradigm and manipulations within it).

By necessity, an interview study uses individual respondents as first-stage sampling units. In the present study they were sampled by the simple random sampling procedure (with complementary address sampling and substitution procedures) described in Chapter 3 (see "Selection of the Interview Sample"). As reported in Appendix A, this first-stage sample satisfactorily reflected the population of the community on several demographic variables. The violence episodes of this study were the second-stage, *systematically sampled* units. The systematic characteristic of this sampling was the selection of the most recent event in a potential series of events for inclusion. This type of second-stage sampling cannot, of course, in any way be considered a procedure for selecting a random sample or any form of probability sample of events or individuals in events. Thus no population estimates can directly be made that would apply to the universe of violent situations occurring in the city during a specific time period or to the universe of violent conflicts experienced by city residents (whether in Thunder Bay itself or elsewhere). Strictly speaking, estimation possibilities were limited to the universe of most recent experiences by individuals living in the community of encounters in which at least they (and in many cases also their antagonists) were victimized by one or more acts of physical violence. Considering the dearth of analytical material in the study of alcohol's connections with aggression and violence, these data can still provide a considerable increment in knowledge.

Some comparisons between the interview study samples of violence episodes and the 1-year police census of violent crime events are also presented and discussed in this chapter. Although the two samples of events are not strictly comparable, such comparisons may provide tentative insights into processes at work in the selection of samples of violence for official recording. From the phenomenological perspective of community residents, these two types of sources—personal experiences and (publicized) episodes of criminal violence—probably combine to create their perception of the extent and causes of violence in the community and society at large. Some conjoint analyses may be justified also on this score.

All interviewees who reported having been subjected to one or more acts of violence since the age of 15 were asked about their most recent victimization. Altogether, 492 respondents out of the 933 interviewed reported that they had been subjected to violence since the age of 15. Out of these, 28 could not remember what incident was the most recent one, 22 could not remember the specific incident in enough detail to allow any analyses, and 7 refused to describe this episode for personal reasons. A total of 57 victims, 37 males and 20 females, made up this internal attrition.[1] The remaining 435 incidents of violence form the basis of the analyses to follow. Weighting for the underrepresentation of women resulted in a weighted total of 452 incidents of physical violence.

Based on these figures, 60% of male and 44% of female city residents reported having been victimized since the age of 15 by some type of violent act (52% of the total weighted sample). Fifty-eight percent of community residents reported having been subjected to either

1. There are some additional missing data on specific variables. This means that the sample sizes vary somewhat from one table to the next. Instead of a tedious repetition of the reasons for this, I give the reasons only with respect to the most central of variables when these are first brought up.

physical violence *or* threats of such violence since the age of 15 (67% of men and 49% of women).

In addition to the difference in sampling procedures, the police reports only included violent incidents that took place within the city limits, whereas some of the most recent experiences of violence reported on in the survey occurred outside this area. Moreover, the former sample was limited to a specific 1-year calendar period, whereas the latter sample was indefinite as to calendar period. As we will see, although there was a clustering in more recent years the range was very wide, with the most distant occasions stretching back 30 years and more.

Some violent incidents had happened before the respondent moved to the city, and others had occurred during a temporary absence from home (in connection with studies in another community, on a trip, etc.). Still others had occurred before the respondents emigrated to Canada, some had occurred during a vacation, and a few had occurred while the respondents were stationed abroad during a war. Experiences directly linked to warfare, such as being wounded in combat, were not included; however, wartime experiences in civilian settings were (e.g., when a soldier on furlough got into a fight over a girl in a dance hall). In all, 72% of the violence reported had occurred within the limits of the city proper, 84% in the province of Ontario, and 93% in Canada.

Close to 60% of the most recent violence to community residents had occurred during the 1970s (i.e., during approximately the last 8 years preceding the interview). Almost 40% had occurred during 3 to 4 years preceding the interview. Eighty percent had occurred within the last 20 years. Analyses showed that there were no significant differences in the nature of the violence that had occurred during different calendar year periods.

The proportion of relatively recent victimizations (within about 8 years of the interview) was greater among women (67%) than among men (53%; $\chi^2 = 8.84$; $df = 1$; $p < .01$). Men seemed to be more likely than women to have had their last experience of physical victimization in their youth; by contrast, women were probably subjected to violence later as well, in their marriages and to some extent in other stable relationships with men. I cannot, however, rule out the possibility that violence generally directed against women had increased during the last few years preceding the survey, and that this was also reflected in this finding.

As might be expected, a larger proportion of the more recent incidents of violence occurred in the community. About 85% of the episodes that had taken place during the previous 8 years had occurred within the city limits, while this was true for only 54% of older incidents. In a few analyses below, I have used as a control sample the

222 events of physical subjections to violent acts that occurred in the city itself within about 8 years of the interviews. This has been done in order to assess, in a rough way, possible effects of including episodes far removed in time. This subsample made up about half the violent events accessed through the survey.

CHARACTERISTICS OF VIOLENCE REPORTED IN THE INTERVIEWS AND IN THE POLICE CENSUS

Information on some aspects of the violent crimes reported to the police, mostly information about assailants, was missing to a greater extent than in the episodes of violence that were accessed through the interview survey. In most regards, these gaps in the data were not large enough to endanger the usefulness of the comparisons to any crippling extent. However, it is evident that police clearance rates are extremely important in assessing the potential extent of bias in the information from police records, including estimates of alcohol involvement.

In comparing the violent crime data with the most recent aggression episodes reported by community residents, I have consistently left out occurrences in which the victims were under the age of 15 and the offenders were under the age of 12 (the criteria used for inclusion in the interview study). This corrective exclusion assumes that the respondents in the survey would invariably have been labeled the victims if the incidents had come to the attention of the police and been entered into their records. This, in all probability, is not the case. However, it is almost assuredly closer to the truth than the alternative assumption that the respondents would in all cases have been labeled suspects or offenders. The truth lies somewhere in between, and either assumption would lead to largely the same exclusions of episodes, since when an offender is a child the victim is also likely to be very young.

Gender of Victims and Assailants

A predominant pattern emerging from numerous studies is that women are the victims in a large proportion of violent crime. For example, about 24% of the victims of homicide in Wolfgang's (1958) study of 588 homicides in Philadelphia during the period 1948–1952 were women, and a Statistics Canada study (1976) showed that 39.5% of victims (and 11.6% of offenders) in homicides committed in Canada during the period 1961 to 1974 were women ($n = 4{,}656$). Calculations on the basis of published findings in the 1982 Canadian Urban Victimization Study show that the proportion of female victimizations out of all victimizations in seven urban centers was 36% (Solicitor General Canada, 1985a). The results of the present interview survey (reported in Chapter 4, "Male and Female Rates of Victimization") showed that approximately half of all victimizations in the community during a 12-month period were directed against women, by this study's comparatively inclusive criteria for violence.

In the police records of the study community, almost half of the victims were female (47%—calculated from Table 5.1). In the most recent victimization episodes reported in the interviews, this share was somewhat lower, 40%.[2] Collapsing the findings of Table 5.1 also makes it possible to summarize the proportions of violent incidents with a female assailant. These made up 16% of the interview episodes and 8% of the violent crimes.

The high proportion of female victims in the police census of violent crimes may reflect the concentration of repeated, very serious violence among a relatively small proportion of women. This fact would not emerge in the analysis of individual episodes in the interview sample, since each respondent was only represented by one episode. There is also an indication in these results that incidents in which a man was victimized by a woman may have been reported to the police to a lesser extent than other incidents: 8% of victimizations in the interview survey were of this nature, whereas only 3% of violent crimes in the police census had this gender constellation. A weak tendency in the same direction can be noted for violence in which a woman was victimized by another woman.

Age of Victims

Table 5.1 also shows the ages of the victims in the two samples of violence. In the retrospectively sampled episodes from the interview survey, the ages naturally refer to the ages of the respondents at the time of the incidents. Both distributions showed a high concentration in young age groups. This could to some extent be expected from the earlier finding on victimizations during the 12 months preceding the interview (see Chapter 4) that young individuals were much more likely to have experienced aggression in various forms. The similarities in age

2. In the results from the interview survey, the respondents are persistently labeled "victims" for the sake of convenience. In some violent crimes this labeling is also somewhat arbitrary. The existence of victim precipitation in some cases (e.g., the victim's initiation of physically violent acts) should be kept in mind; it should also be remembered that the designation "victim" in police reports actually refers to the person on whose behalf a complaint was made.

TABLE 5.1. Characteristics of Violence Episodes Reported in the Interview Survey and in the 1-Year Police Census of Violent Crimes

Characteristic	Victimizations reported in interviews	Violent crimes reported to police during 12 months
Gender of victim and assailant	(n = 450)	(n = 749)
Male victim, male assailant	52%	49%
Male victim, female assailant	8%	3%
Female victim, male assailant	32%	44%
Female victim, female assailant	8%	5%
Age of victim	(n = 448)	(n = 689)
Under 20	24%	24%
20–29	39%	32%
30–39	18%	17%
40–49	10%	14%
50–59	7%	8%
60 and over	2%	5%
Location of episode	(n = 452)	(n = 596)
Own home	34%	[a]
Other home	10%	47%[a]
Work or school	15%	2%
Public drinking place	17%	9%
Street or park	14%	28%
Some other location	10%	14%
Number of participants	(n = 451)	(n = 762)
More than one assailant	14%	18%
More than one victim	n.a.	8%
Relationship of victim to assailant	(n = 436)	(n = 687)
Spouse	21%	23%
Parent, child, sibling, or other relative	11%	7%
Acquaintance or friend	39%	44%
Stranger	28%	26%

Note. Percentages in some categories do not total 100% because of roundings.
[a]No distinction could be made between violent crime occurrences that had occurred in a victim's home and in other private homes, and the figure refers to the sum for these locations.

distributions between the interview study sample and the occurrences of violent crime are remarkable, considering the differences in sampling procedures.

The assailants showed a very similar age concentration among youths (data not shown). As with the age distribution of victims, there was also an almost perfect fit between the violent crime census and the survey sample of violence. (This provides us with a small measure of intuitive faith in the generalizability of findings from the systematically selected sample onto the population of incidents occurring in specific time periods, although this was not a principal purpose of this study.) *Both* the victim and the assailant were under the age of 30 in 52% of the interview survey data and in 43% of the violent crimes. At least one of the participants was under 30 in about three-quarters of both types of episodes. The overrepresentation of youths is a finding that has been replicated in numerous studies of criminal violence in various jurisdictions and in many countries (e.g., Aromaa, 1977b; Central Bureau of Statistics, Sweden, 1981; Ferracuti & Newman, 1974; Goodman et al., 1986; McClintock, 1963, 1975; Solicitor General, Canada, 1983; Wolfgang, 1958).

For reasons specified earlier, incidents in which victims were under the age of 15 and/or offenders were under the age of 12 have been omitted in order to make the selection criteria comparable between the two samples. Thus, the figures on violent crimes underestimate to some degree the proportion of occurrences of violence reported to the police that involved individuals under the age of 30. However, the true figures for violent crimes differ little from those reported above: If these children are included in the analysis, 48% of violent crimes had both participants under the age of 30 (cf. 43%), and 75% had at least one participant under that age (cf. 72%).

Locations of Violence

In Table 5.1, the locations in which the violent events occurred are also shown. Although a private home was the most common location for both types of events, there were substantial differences in the proportions of incidents that occurred in other locales. Outdoor public areas were more common in the violence that came to the attention of the police, whereas the workplace or school was reported much more often in the interviews. Public drinking places were reported as the site of violence about twice as often in the interview survey episodes. This may indicate that public drinking places are relatively high-risk locations, especially for male members of the *general* population.

I have already speculated about the different locations in which men and women experience aggression. In the interview survey data, there were considerable differences between men and women in the prevalence of their own homes as the location for victimizations by violence: 17% of men (n = 270) and 60% of women (n = 182) were last victimized in their own homes.

By contrast, relatively little violence reported in the interviews had taken place in a private home other than a respondent's own, and there were very small differences between men and women in the relative frequency of this location as the scene of both types of episodes. Table 5.2 shows the proportions of male and female victims who were subjected to violence in different locations. Collapsing all private homes into one category for the interview survey enables these data to be compared with those from the violent crime census. The share of violence in a home setting was very high among women in both sets of data (73% in the interviews and 65% in the police data). By comparison, slightly more than one-fourth of male victimizations had taken place in a private home. The share of violent encounters that took place at work or at school differed greatly between men and women; the same was true for public drinking establishments. The difference between genders was considerable for police-attended violent incidents occurring in streets, parks, and the like, but not for physical violence in such locations reported in the interviews.

The prevalence of public drinking places as locations for victimizations of the men in the community was particularly high in the data from the interview study: About one-quarter of men had last been victimized in this location. I have noted earlier (see Chapter 4) that a high share of men had witnessed violent behavior in public drinking establishments during a 12-month period. It would be wrong, of course, to attribute all violence in taverns and bars to drinking alone. In many cases, social and interactional processes that increase the likelihood of aggression may occur in these locales, largely independently of any alcohol effects on mind and behavior. In other cases (and these are probably in the majority), alcohol effects interact with social, psychological, and situational factors. These combined effects then lead to in-

TABLE 5.2. Proportion of Violence Episodes Reported in the Interview Survey and in the 1-Year Police Census of Violent Crimes That Occurred in Various Settings, by Gender of the Victim

	Victimizations reported in interviews		Violent crimes reported to police during 12 months	
Location	Male victims (n = 270)	Female victims (n = 182)	Male victims (n = 292)	Female victims (n = 304)
Private home	26%	73%	28%	65%
Work or school	22%	6%	2%	1%
Public drinking place	24%	5%	12%	7%
Street or park	16%	11%	40%	18%
Some other location	12%	6%	18%	10%

Note. Percentages in some categories do not total 100% because of rounding.

creased risks of conflict and aggressive encounters. These interactions deserve empirical study and theoretical analysis as much as any direct effects of alcohol in the blood on risk of aggression.

Violent crimes in a public drinking place occurred disproportionately often after midnight. Physically violent encounters in drinking places reported in the survey took place much less often in that time period. The most common locale for violence during all periods of the day was the home. In addition to violence within the walls of taverns and bars, a substantial proportion occurred just outside drinking places, in the street, in a parking lot, or in a backyard. This occurred very often around closing time, when scattered observations in the city also indicated that vandalism (e.g., damage to parked cars) was likely to occur.

There are strong indications in the results presented in Table 5.2 that work and school locations were underrepresented as sites of violence in the violent crime data, especially among men. The same can be said for male victimizations in drinking establishments, whereas women seemed to receive better official coverage when victimized in such locations.

The locations included in the residual category of "some other locations" were very varied, and none of them were prevalent enough or of sufficient interest to warrant separate tabulations. Among the ones represented in the two sets of data were stores, malls or plazas, hotels and motels, stadiums and arenas, buses and private cars, summer cottages, a theater, a church, a grain elevator, a bowling alley, a drive-in theater, a military installation, a restaurant not licensed to serve alcohol, a car wash, a laundromat, an unemployment office, a welfare office, a credit union office, a hospital, a jail, and a family court.

Number of Participants

In a number of violent incidents, the respondents/victims in the interview survey had to face more than one assailant (i.e., the answer to the question "Did more than one person hurt you?" was affirmative). In these cases, the respondents were asked to select the most active individual among these in describing the adversary. This was done mainly for economy in data collection and analyses. More than one assailant was involved in 14% of the violent situations reported in the interviews and 18% of violent crime incidents in the police census. As might be expected on the basis of the differences in the locations where violence had occurred, men were much more likely to have been victimized by multiple assailants: The proportion in the interview survey was 20% for men, compared to 7% for women ($\chi^2 = 13.23$, $df = 1$, $p < .001$). In violent crimes, fully 28% of men had been assaulted by more than one assailant, while only 8% of women had ($\chi^2 = 40.14$, $df = 1$, $p < .0001$). In all probability, this difference mainly reflects a higher share of domestic aggression and violence within close relationships among women. Age at the time of the incident was generally inversely related to the probability of having more than one adversary; this fits in with stereotypes concerning a higher incidence of group violence in youth.

In addition to episodes of violence in which there was more than one assailant, there were a number of events in which the respondents were aided by other individuals. In the interview survey, data on these were available only in (often less than complete) brief open-ended descriptions of the events. For the violent crime census, on the other hand, there was systematically recorded information on whether more than one person was designated as a victim; this was the case in 8% of the crime incidents.

Relationships of Victims to Assailants

An acquaintance or friend was the most common adversary in both types of episodes, with prevalences around 40% (see Table 5.1). The distributions of prevalences for different relationships in the two sets of data differed relatively little. As expected, marital violence made up a much larger share of the victimizations of women than of men—another of the patterns found almost universally in human violence (e.g., Gelles, 1987; Germain, Mattila, Meyers-Törnroth, & Polkunen-Gartz, 1980; Solicitor General, Canada, 1985a; Strauss, Gelles, & Steinmetz, 1980). In physical violence reported in the interview survey, 41% of women had their husbands as their assailants in the most recent episode, whereas men had last been victimized physically by their wives in only 7% of these events. The most common situation in which a man was subjected to some physical acts of violence was an encounter with a total stranger (36%), followed by episodes involving different types of acquaintances (e.g., a person from work or school in 22% of the episodes, a person known mainly from the neighborhood in 12%). Combining all family violence (i.e., spouses, parents, children and other relatives) results in a proportion of 13% family violence in the victimizations of men and 61% in those of women.

If we take into account the fact that some of the respondents had never been married (and thus did not belong to the population at risk for marital conflict), we get a more representative picture for marital violence. Of ever-married women who had been subjected to physical violence since the age of 15, over half (52%) had been victimized by their spouses in their most recent event of physical violence. For men, the corresponding figure was 8%. It is also interesting to note the difference in total family-involved violence for the single (never-married) respondents, compared to ever-married men and women. Single women had been victimized in family conflict in 18% of their most recent subjections to violent acts ($n = 33$), while this was the case for only 3% of single males ($n = 58$). Ever-married women had this experience in 70% of the cases ($n = 142$), compared to 17% of ever-married men ($n = 203$).

It should be pointed out that these proportions for most recent episodes tell us nothing about the *rate* of, for instance, victimizations in marital violence among married men. If we were to base our interpretations *solely* on what we know from the survey data on most recent victimizations, we might conclude that married men may be victimized by their wives as often as married women are subjected to violent acts by their husbands. This is logically possible because the lower prevalence in the most recent events could be due to the fact that married men are much more likely *also* to be involved in violence at work, in taverns, and so forth, so that victimizations in marital violence (although as common as among married women) may be "overshadowed" by violence in other relationships. It is only when we put our findings in the context of other findings from this study, such as the rates of victimizations among men and women during the last 12 months (see Chapter 4, where it is noted that the incidence of victimization by violence over this time span was equal between men and women in the city), as well as findings in similar studies (e.g., Solicitor General, Canada, 1985a; Statistics Canada, 1976), that we can assess this possibility as being totally unlikely. I mention this only in order to point out once again the special nature of the samples of most recent events, so as to prevent the wrong kind of conclusions from an exclusive reliance on this type of sample. Combined with the incidence data on subjection to physical violence during the last 12 months (and to some extent with the data from the violent crime census), there should remain no doubt that victimization in family violence was much more common among women than among men in this community.

In the context of marital violence, it is also worth noting that among women who had not yet married, the share of physical violence committed by a boyfriend was 21%. In comparison, 9% of never-married men were most recently subjected to violence by their girlfriends ($p > .20$). The share of violent encounters between strangers seems to be determined more by gender than by marital status. Single women were victimized by somebody at work or school much more often than married women; their victimizations in these settings approached the levels of men.

The findings from the police census of violent crimes support the picture given by the interview survey's systematic samples of events. Among female victims, the husbands were the offenders in 37% of the cases. This was on the same order of magnitude as for the survey sample of violence. Among male victims of violent crime, their wives were the offenders in only 3% of incidents. The total share of family violence in violent crimes was 45% for female victims and only 9% among male victims.

The category "acquaintance or friend" includes a wide variety of different kinds of relationships. In addition to the special nature of such relationships in "skid row" and other "lower-class" bars (to be discussed in some detail below), an "acquaintance" in the world of the average citizen can be someone whom a person sees and associates with at work every day, or a person who is seen only about once a month at the corner grocery, where nods or a few words are exchanged. Differences in familiarity and related interaction patterns are naturally of central importance in the genesis of issues of conflict and in the escalation of conflict into open aggression.

For the episodes of physical violence in the interview survey, systematic information was obtained on how well a victim knew his/her adversary (see question 18 in Appendix B). This question was only asked if the antagonist was not a member of the respondent's family. It was assumed that the respondent knew an adversary from his/her own family or a relative "very well." Table 5.3 provides a look at patterns of familiarity in violence between nonrelatives as related to the gender of the victim. It is clear that women were more likely than men to have been victimized by someone whom they knew well, even when relatives and family members are omitted from consideration. The difference between the genders in the proportion of nonrelated assailants who were very well known was highly significant ($\chi^2 = 17.06$, $df = 1$, $p < .001$). Correspondingly, men more commonly par-

TABLE 5.3. Familiarity of the Assailant in the Most Recent Episodes of Physical Violence by Gender of Victim (Family Members and Relatives Not Included)

Extent to which victim knew assailant	Male victims ($n = 240$)	Female victims ($n = 86$)	Total ($n = 326$)
Very well	16%	37%	22%
Fairly well	18%	21%	19%
A little	14%	5%	11%
Hardly at all	11%	9%	11%
Not at all	41%	28%	37%

ticipated in violent conflict with total strangers. The distributions differed at a statistically highly significant level ($\chi^2 = 21.02$, $df = 4$, $p < .001$).

Summary

The findings from this comparison of the interview survey data and the police census data can be briefly summarized as follows. Young age and family relationships predominated in the serious aggression occurring among the residents of the city, as in most other populations that have been studied. Especially when women were involved in aggression, they most often had other family members as their adversaries. In addition, even when women participated in aggression outside the family, this tended to occur more often in close relationships than was the case for men. Men were much more likely to be victimized by strangers and in public settings.

RELATIONSHIPS AND ISSUES IN TAVERN VIOLENCE

General aggression, and the use of and encounters with physical force, are far from unitary phenomena throughout the life cycle of an individual. Depending on the age of adversaries, different relationships are typically involved in conflict, and these occur in different types of settings and social contexts. The reasons for conflict differ with the different patterns of relationship, as well as the locations and social contexts in which conflict occurs. The social meaning and the transactional symbolism inherent in the aggressive acts will also differ according to such factors. Again, we should ask how alcohol use by one or both participants in these situations will affect the general symbolism of actions in conflict and of the consequences of these actions, as well as the situational and individual interpretations of that symbolism.

For the purpose of explicating the different roles played by alcohol use, alcohol use settings, users of alcohol, and so on in human violence, correlative data on violence that occurs in public drinking places are of central interest. They are of special value insofar as they point to the social dynamics of some alcohol-related violence. Convergent theoretical backgrounds are provided by several excellent studies on the behavior patterns and normative expectations of such settings, as well as the individual and societal needs served by these establishments (e.g., Anderson, 1978; Cavan, 1966; Roebuck & Frese, 1976). These are helpful in the study of conflict dynamics, but they have to be integrated with known effects of alcohol. Such an attempt (as well as attempts at theoretically integrating known effects of alcohol with the dynamics of violent behavior, conflict issues, etc., in domestic violence) has to be left for the future, however. The discussion here is concerned solely with taking a social, dynamic, and relational perspective on alcohol-related violence by way of illustrations from observations made in public drinking places.

Violent crimes reported in the 1-year police census, and violent encounters reported in the interview survey, showed somewhat differing patterns with regard to the frequency of various relationships between adversaries in public drinking settings. Few marital violence situations occurred in drinking establishments, according to both sources; only 2% of episodes from both data sources were of this nature. Other family relationships had approximately the same (lack of) magnitude. However, there was a very high proportion of violence between acquaintances or friends in tavern or bar settings in the violent crime material (75%; $n = 60$), whereas this share was much smaller in the episodes reported in the interviews (33%; $n = 66$). The difference was significant at the .001 level ($\chi^2 = 20.27$, $df = 1$). Instead, most of the tavern violence reported by the community residents occurred between total strangers (63%).

The violence in public drinking establishments that comes to the attention of the police probably stems to a large extent from conflicts within marginal subgroups of the community. These subgroups frequent special drinking places that cater to lower social strata. The patrons include a comparatively high proportion of individuals with various types of drinking problems. This was revealed in the observations in public drinking establishments that were carried out concurrently with the interview survey, and it was also evident from the scanty descriptions provided in the police census data. In such settings there is a great deal of "market" interaction (selling merchandise, attempting to borrow money, asking somebody for a drink or a cigarette, etc.); Cavan (1966) mentions the selling of stolen goods in what she calls the "marketplace bar." In connection with these activities there is a great deal of milling around, as well as several additional varieties of tension that do not exist in most other types of drinking establishments. The "market" character and the tensions are reinforced by the fact that these establishments also serve as locations where members of the opposite sex can be picked up. Again, Cavan (1966) mentions the arrangement of "commercial sex" transactions as a feature of bars of this sort.

The commodities and services supplied and demanded in the bars of the lowest strata are typically rather unassuming. In one incident I describe in more detail later (see Chapter 9), two patrons offered their Christmas ham for sale in order to get more money for beer. Another sequence of interaction from the tavern observations also illustrates the type of marginal "market" behavior that would be unheard of in most other types of drinking establishments.

> A male patron in his 40s had been seen by the observers about 3 weeks earlier in another tavern. At that time he told the observers that he needed $1.85 for a phone call because he had car trouble. The observers gave him some money, but had seen him since asking for money. Now, he tried to get a similar sum of money from one of the other patrons observed; the patron refused.

In the following observational sequence, something besides small change was at stake.

> A heavily intoxicated man carrying a suitcase and a bag was asking patrons at every table whether they would take him home with them. He asked the observers, but they declined. One of the patrons at a table being observed saw him coming and waved him off. A woman sitting at the same table called the man with the suitcase a "creep." Even an elderly man sitting at the same table, who was quite drunk and could hardly keep his head up, put his head in his hands and said "No, no, no, no, no!" in response to the request.

Behavior linked to the "sexual marketplace" character of some taverns can lead to violent conflict. Old sex-related wrongdoings or negative reputations are openly brought out when a suitable state of intoxication has been reached, as in the following extended sequence.

> A young girl who did not look more than 16 years old, dressed in very dirty-looking jeans and boots, seemed very intoxicated. She had been walking around looking for trouble. One man walked over to her and said something to her while she was sitting at a table. The girl (whom I will call Sue) pushed her chair out and started yelling at him: "Where's Margaret, where's Margaret!" She then pushed the man and said, "Come on, come on, I'll fight you!", but he turned his back and walked back to his table.
>
> Sue turned to another man and said, "What have you got to say?". The man just smiled and laughed, which seemed to infuriate her: "Come on, you want to fight a whore? I'll fight you!" She went up to him and gave him a couple of punches. He did not respond. She then knocked him right off his chair onto the floor. He got up and sat down. All the people in the bar were watching. Sue threw her jacket off and repeated, "Come on, I'll fight you!" Both the man she had punched and the first man just looked away. At that point a third man, who had been playing pool, came over and tried to act as a peacemaker. He picked up her jacket from the floor and talked to her reassuringly. Sue finally smiled, put her jacket on, and left the bar.
>
> The peace was short-lived: Sue returned 2 minutes later, threw her jacket to still another man, and then pushed him in the back. He began shouting at her: "You race me, you race me!" The men in the bar were laughing at her, and she became really angry. The peacemaker again came over to her, as did the waitress; they tried to calm her down. The man led

Sue to a chair and put her down there. She started kicking and biting. The chair tipped over and she fell down on the floor. Her uncle seemed to be in the bar, because she started saying, "Uncle, uncle, that guy raped me!" The uncle looked at the peacemaker and asked him whether he really raped her. The peacemaker just threw an arm up in the air and walked away. Sue sat in her chair repeating, "You raped me, you raped me."

A few minutes later Sue sat down at her uncle's table, from which she continued her accusations. The uncle asked her, "Why don't you keep quiet and go sit somewhere else if you want to cause trouble?" Ignoring him, Sue went on with her accusations against the peacemaker, richly interspersed with profanity (e.g., "You fucker"). Her uncle told her, "Go somewhere else if you want trouble. Go find another bar." Sue got up, put her jacket on, and went to the other section of the tavern. There she pushed a man from behind and said, "Your friend raped me!" He replied that he did not know the man and went over to the pool table to play. Sue gave him a kick in the rear end and grabbed his sweater so that his pool partner had to release him. The partner pulled her away and said, "Come on, leave him alone. You had enough of that." Sue just kept going on and on. Finally the man she was grabbing said, "You get off my fucking back or I'll nail you." That seemed to shake her up a bit. All the other people started laughing. He shook her loose, faced her, and repeated, "Get off my back." Sue did not seem to know what to say. She walked away swearing and got her coat from where she had left it at an empty table.

One of the women in the bar then shouted at Sue, "You're nothing but a dumb whore. Why don't you shut up and get out of here?" Sue started yelling back, and the woman challenged her: "You want to fight? I'll fight you!" Sue yelled back, took her coat, and walked toward the exit. Just as she was almost at the door, the bartender came running after her; he seemed to have had just about enough. Sue picked up an ashtray from a table near the exit, turned around, and seemed ready to throw it at someone. The bartender reached her, grabbed her arm and wrapped it around her, got her to the door, took the ashtray out of her hand, and literally threw her out the door. Sue grabbed the handle of the door, and the bartender began pushing her down the stairs on the outside and gave her a couple of kicks. Finally, she was outside. After a minute or so, she stuck her head in and shouted, "I'm going to call the police on all you fuckers!"

After about 10 minutes Sue returned through the back door. She was quieter and just walked around looking at everybody. They ignored her completely. The bartender seemed to have called the police. Someone warned Sue that the police were on their way; they arrived about 2 minutes later. Customers pointed the police in the direction where Sue was last seen. They went to the bartender and looked around for Sue, but she seemed to have exited from the other section of the bar. A couple of drunken patrons stopped the police to talk to them and shake their hands. Two other officers came in through the back door and just watched. The first two officers moved toward the back, and a man waved them over. They

> went to see him, and he struggled out of his chair and put out his hand to shake their hands. They just smiled and nodded. All the policemen then left the bar.

The behavior of the witnesses to this interaction is perhaps just as telling as the behavior of the main actors. Although this could hardly be considered a "standing pattern of behavior" (Cavan, 1966) in this and other similar establishments, the interaction indicates that both the management's and the patron's tolerance level for aggression and other angry behavior was very high (although it was finally exceeded in this incident). It is also a conceptually sobering thought that in standard coding schemes the relationships between most of the adversaries in this violence would probably have been coded as those of "acquaintances" or "friends." Still, the issues differ when patrons know each other, and so do the dynamics. In some cases, drinking places are identity-defining forums and places where self-esteem is sought (e.g., Anderson, 1978; Cavan, 1966; Macrory, 1952; Roebuck & Frese, 1976); as I argue in another context, it is often found with the partial aid of alcohol. In such settings, more is at stake in conflict and general interaction, since statuses, rights, and identities are defined that carry over from one night to the next. Sue's challenge to the others to "fight a whore" indicates that she was putting her assigned status on the line and wanted to redefine it by means of violence as a status-defining activity.

Strangers are often adversaries in the physical aggression that occurs in public drinking places, no doubt in part because there are disproportionately many people present in these settings who do not know each other from before. In the present study's tavern observations, as well as in an analysis of the dynamics of specific episodes of violence reported in the interview survey, it was found that there was a strong ingroup aspect to a substantial proportion of the aggression occurring between strangers or near-strangers in drinking establishments. One patron would be (by someone's definition) wronged, and the whole drinking group would stand up to his defense. In such an ingroup situation, escalation into physical violence is more likely than in individual confrontations, since only one of the actors usually has to exceed the boundary beyond which "things get out of hand." It is possible that cognitive alcohol effects potentiate causal processes linked to regular crowd or group behavior. (Central aspects of, e.g., soccer hooliganism are probably better understood through alcohol effects interacting with social processes.) The following example from the news media is an extreme instance of tavern-related crowd behavior and the apparent effectiveness of structuring a situation as an ingroup–outgroup confrontation (again probably aided by general effects of alcohol):

> PETIT ROCHER, [New Brunswick] (CP)—About 300 angry village residents exchanged shots with two or three members of a local motorcycle gang before the mob destroyed a large clubhouse, two small camps, a pick-up truck, two cars and five motorcycles last night.
>
> A village official, who refused to be identified, said a jeering crowd of more than 1000 confronted some members of the Daltons motorcycle club earlier yesterday at a tavern and challenged them to fight.
>
> The gang members refused to fight with the crowd which included about 50 men with guns and several others carrying baseball bats. The motorcyclists fled to their isolated clubhouse in woods about five miles from here.
>
> The crowd followed and gunfire was exchanged before the gang members fled into the woods and the clubhouse was burned. A dog owned by a gang member was killed.
>
> Two Royal Canadian Mounted Police [RCMP] officers were injured lightly by flying glass when they arrived at the burning clubhouse and the back window of one police car was shattered. The cause was not known.
>
> "It's still not determined what happened," said Staff Sergeant George Gauthier of the RCMP detachment in Bathurst. "Things are still pretty confused around here."
>
> He said police had been aware since late Sunday that trouble was brewing after a fight in a tavern sent two men to hospital and injured three others. . . .
>
> The official said the crowd, many of whom had been drinking, decided to pursue the motorcyclists, who left the tavern, after one of the men injured in Sunday's fight arrived at the crowded bar. He had been thrown out of a window and suffered a face wound which required 50 stitches to close.
>
> "When they saw him, that was it." . . . (*Toronto Star*, August 30, 1978)

In an earlier illustration of tavern violence (see Chapter 1, pp. 7–8), the brawl also continued outside the premises. This is a very common pattern. Sometimes the antagonists themselves decide to enact a definitive resolution to the conflict somewhere outside, where they are less likely to be stopped by other patrons or a bouncer; at other times they are ejected and left to seek a resolution somewhere else if they so wish.

Ritualized or merely structured aspects of actions in a setting—in this case, drunken brawls in taverns—are related to the stereotypes that people have of these actions, in a form of bidirectional determination. No doubt structured violent behavior in these settings gives rise to the stereotypical perceptions of "barroom brawls." On the other hand, such stereotypes also to some extent foster the phenomenon itself. Entering a melee in a bar, stepping outside to conclude the proceedings, coming back next weekend to decide who really is the king of the turf, and the like are to some extent products of social stereotyping and not just a sum of individual motivations. Such are the semiotics of this type of human violence, and similar patterns of determination occur in other types of violence. In this way human violence is a guided activity, although we would expect alcohol to leave its natural-level imprints on the processes and outcomes of this activity.

6

The Presence of Alcohol in Episodes of Violence

Violent crimes have formed the almost exclusive source of natural aggression episodes in the systematic study of alcohol use by adversaries in aggression. As a consequence, available empirical findings on alcohol's role in naturally occurring aggression have been sifted through the largely idiosyncratic recording habits of the police or the courts and have also been determined by the reporting tendencies of the populace.[1] Consequently, little information is available on the extent of alcohol use as it relates to central characteristics of the participants and the situational or contextual characteristics in more common types of physical aggression. Even with regard to violent crime, very little is known about some central variables, such as the amounts of alcohol used prior to aggression.

The present study's data on the incidence of violence among community residents during a 12-month period indicate, as have numerous earlier investigations in other populations, that the actual rate of violence is vastly greater than that which comes to the attention of the police (only some cases of which are later processed in the courts). Potential biases introduced by the social and individual processing of violent incidents into this subset cannot be disregarded. With the present study's focus on the linkage between alcohol use and aggressive behavior, the potential selective variables of greatest concern are the

1. As noted earlier, studies of autopsy records and some emergency room studies have also been carried out, but these have generally focused on the characteristics of the victim, the nature of injuries, or the like, and have provided little information on the incident of violence itself and the characteristics of other participants, including the assailant.

alcohol use characteristics of one or more participants. Since so much of our meager knowledge of the role of alcohol in violent behavior is based on official crime reports and medical records, it is important to know whether alcohol use is correctly represented in the samples accessed through criminal and medical consequences of violence. The present community data permit this question to be examined to some extent.

Nonrandom selection in the reporting of episodes of interpersonal violence may also affect the information obtained about aggression and alcohol use in any survey based on self-reports. Estimates of the prevalence of aggression may have to be considered minimum estimates in any interview study of this kind, because of deficient sampling frames, social desirability effects, and faulty recall. Still, such estimates in all likelihood give a more valid picture of the patterns of violence in society than do official records of episodes of violence.

The present study tried to overcome some of the shortcomings of officially documented violence by systematically collecting information on the extent and nature of alcohol use in situations where violence occurred. (In addition, data were collected on three different types of drinking occasions. Some results are presented from these in order to compare consumption prior to violence with consumption in more typical drinking episodes.) As I have noted earlier, the interview survey had many of the characteristics of a victimization study, although it differed in the number of details collected about individual episodes, as well as in its emphasis on the use of alcohol.

The nature of the two-stage systematic sampling of episodes and participants in these episodes makes generalizations to even the local universe of violence situations experienced by community residents hazardous. The emphasis in this chapter is instead on comparative analyses between subgroups of the community. In addition to its practicality, the sampling procedure has one important feature, however, which I make use of here and will utilize again later in the cross-national replication: It is a well-defined and replicable type of sampling (as opposed to "seat-of-the-pants" sampling or most purposive sampling). Within random sampling variations, we can expect the findings to be the same if other samples have been drawn from the same population during the same time period, using the same sampling procedure.

ASSESSING THE CHARACTERISTICS OF ALCOHOL USE

Findings pertaining to the presence of alcohol in violence episodes are described in this chapter. I hope that they will give some impetus to further questions regarding the different ways in which alcohol use is related to aggressive behavior and to physical violence. In addition to the standard measure of "total alcohol involvement," which dominates studies of alcohol's role in violent crime (see Chapter 2), some other alcohol use characteristics have been assessed. The amounts consumed before the violence occurred are naturally of central interest to possible explanatory models of aggression in connection with alcohol use. For rather obvious reasons, it was not possible to get detailed information on the use of alcohol by the respondents' assailants. In most cases, the respondents were not in a position to observe the assailants' drinking or to get this information in some other way (e.g., from witnesses). Information on drinking by the assailants is restricted to the respondents' knowledge or assessment of whether the assailants had been drinking prior to the aggressive encounter and whether the assailants were "drunk" (see questions 23 and 24 in Appendix B).

With regard to the respondents' own alcohol use, the interviewers attempted to get as accurate information as possible on the amounts that they had consumed prior to becoming the targets of violent acts (see questions 25 and 26 in Appendix B). In some cases, the information on amounts and types of beverage was more in the nature of an estimate of typical drinking at such occasions, and not based on actual or attempted recall; in most cases, however, the respondents made honest attempts at accurate recall. No independent data were available to indicate just how successful these attempts were. The respondents' typical drinking patterns have not been included in the analyses to follow, since only current drinking patterns could be asked about with any degree of validity, and not those that prevailed at the time when the sampled violent events occurred. Instead, the analyses deal exclusively with questions surrounding the use of alcohol immediately prior to the violence.

As discussed in Appendix A, some checks were carried out to assess the validity of the aggregated responses on alcohol use. Brief questionnaires were sent to some of the attrition cases (mainly refusals), and the interviewers were asked to assess the extent to which the persons they had interviewed showed reluctance or hesitation to answer questions about alcohol use (and about violence). In addition, the effect of the presence of outsiders in the interview was assessed. The results of these checks, although by no means conclusive, showed no great or statistically significant effects on the resultant validity of central information on drinking and on aggression experiences.

In the respondents' assessments of drunkenness of the persons who victimized them, one would under ideal circumstances be able to eliminate the influence of some conditional alcohol factors or alternative referents of "alcohol use," since "being drunk" refers to the end product of all different determinations: the behavior of the drinking individual.

Extraneous effects on blood alcohol concentration (BAC) such as consumption of food, the congener content of the beverage, different drinking speeds, and the like, have in effect been controlled for by using assessments of intoxication instead of amounts consumed. The accuracy of this measure would not meet any high standards, though. The "instrument" is a respondent's perception and definition of a person's being "drunk." These criteria may differ from one subgroup of the population to another, and especially between different cultural or subcultural groups. On the other hand, the attribution itself of a person as being "drunk," and related attributions projected onto the drinker on the basis of this definition in a social situation, to some extent determine behavior directed toward this person and thus also the ensuing interaction. This occurs in part independently of the actual BACs involved. As a general rule, it should be remembered that even when we are dealing with ratio scale measures of the highest possible sophistication, such as measures of BAC, we are in fact dealing concomitantly with other causally active scales that are by no means perfectly correlated with the former ones. These latter scales are socially defined. They are effectual in social interaction, and they are typically discrete and multidimensionally determined. Defining someone as being "drunk" will have effects in the interactional episode beyond the pharmacological effects of alcohol, and these effects will differ from one sociocultural sphere to another.

Information on the drinking of participants in the violent crimes of the city was based on the written occurrence reports of the police over a 12-month period. Drinking by offenders or victims was coded only if there was specific mention of it in the reports. Because there were no specific questions or specific instructions regarding the recording of presence of alcohol in the participants on this occurrence form, all estimates of alcohol involvement from this data source must be considered minimum estimates. (This is the case for most studies on alcohol involvement in officially detected violent crime. In medically attended violence, there are in some cases special personnel present for the purpose of registering and/or measuring the presence of alcohol in victims; e.g., see Cherpitel, 1989.) It was left up to the individual police officers, with their personal idiosyncracies, to include any type of information on drinking by the participants. In consequence, the descriptions of drinking on these forms ranged from the very general to the fairly specific, and touched on several types of alcohol use variables that could have causal relevance for behavior.

Sometimes the apparent state of intoxication of the participants in violent crime, their alcohol-related mood, their capability for task performance, or the actions taken by the police because of the intoxicated state were referred to in such terms as these: "Very drunk," "Drinking but was not drunk," "Was feeling good," "Both in intoxicated state," "Drinking had taken place," "Appeared intoxicated," "Consuming too much liquor," "Impaired," "An odour of alcoholic beverage on his breath," "Either under the influence of alcohol or drugs," "Taken to detox," and the like. Other reports included the amounts consumed by the offenders and/or victims in varying detail: "Had a few drinks," "Couple of beers," "Nine beers in the evening," "Had consumed one bottle of wine," "Several ounces of vodka," "Six double ryes," ". 16 on breathalyzer."

In addition to information on amounts consumed or state of intoxication, an attempt was made to gather information on the length of the drinking prior to the violent crime. The following type of information was available in a few of the occurrence reports: "Drinking greater part of the day," "Day-long drinking spree," "Drinking for 7 hours," "Had been drinking overnight," "Drinking for 4 days," "Drinking for quite some time." In the same way, some scattered information was available on the drinking patterns of the victims or the offenders (e.g., "Heavy drinker") or the type of beverage consumed (e.g., "Drinking beer and wine"). None of this information was systematic enough to provide a base for analyzing the prevalence of different types of alcohol use in connection with the violence that had come to the attention of the police.

Fewer than ten out of the 847 reports on violent crime contained references to (possible) drug use. In the interviews, references to drug use by the assailant were equally rare. There was little general concern about the use of drugs in the city, and even less about hard drugs. The news media hardly paid any attention to drug use or abuse, and this seemed to validly reflect its low prevalence at the time of the study. The study's observers in the taverns and bars of the city reported seeing an occasional patron smoking a "joint" outside, and could smell marihuana smoke in the washrooms in connection with some observational sessions. They also observed a few cases of apparent trafficking, but this seemed to be limited to marihuana, and to locations where youth congregated (especially in connection with live rock concerts).

ALCOHOL INVOLVEMENT IN VIOLENT CRIMES

Drinking by Offenders and Victims: Validity Problems

In a great number of the incidents of criminal violence that came to the attention of the police, it was not recorded in the occurrence reports whether the victims or the suspects/offenders had consumed alcohol prior to the crime, as I have noted above. This lack of information was of course inevitable in the cases where the suspect was not known or apprehended by the police.

There was no direct information available in these data on whether the suspects were known and whether they had been interrogated by the police. Direct estimates cannot therefore be made of the influence of nonclearance on alcohol involvement estimates. However, if it is assumed (rather safely) that the police knew the identity of a suspect if the exact birth date of the suspect was known and recorded in the occurrence report, rough assessments can be made. When the birth date was known, 38% of suspects were recorded as having been drinking, 8% had definitely not used alcohol, and for the remaining 55% the recording police officers did not provide any information on alcohol use by the offenders ($n = 381$). In comparison, when the exact birth date was not recorded, 20% of the offenders were recorded as having used alcohol, 9% had definitely used no alcohol, and for 72% no information on alcohol use was recorded ($n = 462$). In interpreting these findings, it should be kept in mind that the former subsample was probably biased on a number of central variables. There was, for instance, an overrepresentation of cases in which the victim knew the suspect, and among these were the occurrences of domestic violence.

Table 6.1 shows a breakdown of drinking prior to violence by location of the crime and by whether the exact birth dates of the offender and the victim, respectively, were recorded. Occurrence reports in which the birth date of the *victim* was not recorded provide a baseline for police practice of not recording birth date, even though the identity of a participant in violence was known; the subsample of occurrences in which the *offender's* birth date was not recorded can be interpreted as the union of (1) the set of cases in which the offender was unknown and (2) the set of cases in which the offender was known but no note was made of his/her birth date.

Table 6.1 indicates that there was no great difference in alcohol involvement between "known" and "unknown" offenders in domestic violence. Neither was there a difference for victims in domestic cases whose birth date was recorded, as compared to those for whom it was not entered in the report. On the other hand, there were substantial differences between these two types of violent crime samples for other locations.

Knowing the identity of the suspect/offender clearly resulted in more alcohol use being recorded, independently of where the violence took place. Taken together with the lack of real difference in domestic violence, it means that the higher proportion of alcohol use by the offender (and victim) in incidents in which the suspect/offender was definitely known to the police was not totally occasioned by a dispropor-

TABLE 6.1. Drinking by Offender and Victim in Violent Crimes that Occurred in Various Locations, as Related to Whether the Offender's and Victim's Exact Birth Dates Were Recorded by the Police

	Drinking by offender when date of birth was:		Drinking by victim when date of birth was:	
Location	Recorded	Not recorded	Recorded	Not recorded
Private home	39% ($n = 207$)	35% ($n = 149$)	22% ($n = 242$)	20% ($n = 104$)
Public drinking place	50% ($n = 28$)	35% ($n = 49$)	61% ($n = 59$)	22% ($n = 18$)
Street or park	38% ($n = 93$)	11% ($n = 172$)	27% ($n = 203$)	19% ($n = 62$)
Other location	25% ($n = 53$)	5% ($n = 92$)	16% ($n = 99$)	15% ($n = 46$)
Total	38% ($n = 381$)	20% ($n = 462$)	26% ($n = 613$)	19% ($n = 230$)

tionately high level of (known) alcohol involvement in events occurring in private homes and close relationships, although this certainly had some effect.

Obviously, because the identity of a proportion of offenders was not known to the police, there was an underestimation of alcohol use in the violent crime data of the community. The fact that the victims' recorded drinking was also affected by whether or not a victim's birth date was recorded (although to a much lesser extent) indicates that idiosyncratic recording habits probably also in part determined the pattern for recorded alcohol use of offenders. That is, an officer who was conscientious enough to record the exact birth date of a victim might also be conscientious enough to record information on his/her alcohol use, and the same pattern probably existed for the information on offenders. A number of potentially confounding factors should be introduced as test factors for added confidence in these interpretations, but this would take us too far afield into purely methodological considerations. Still, these are very central questions when police reports are used for the assessment of alcohol use prior to violence.

The incidents that occurred in settings other than a private home clearly include more missing information on the suspects' drinking. Were we to generalize information on the suspects' drinking from the events in which the suspects' identity was definitely known, we would arrive at a rate of 38% drinking by offenders/suspects. This compares to the estimate of 28% for all violent crime events (see below).

The low rates of recorded alcohol use in public drinking places should also be noted, especially for cases in which birth date was not recorded. No acceptable corrective procedure is available for the cases of "alcohol use not known," and estimates of the statistical share of alcohol in this violent crime census must thus be considered minimum estimates. The cases for which information on alcohol use was not recorded are treated here as cases in which alcohol had not been used, since estimates of alcohol involvement are based on the total base figures, including the "not knowns." This is a standard procedure in studies estimating the share of drinking in violent crimes, and is done in order to preclude any positive bias (e.g., Amir, 1971; Gibson, Linden, & Johnson, 1980; Statistics Canada, 1976; Wolfgang, 1958). The procedure leaves a great deal of room for effects of idiosyncratic recording practices in different jurisdictions and countries. These naturally affect estimates of alcohol involvement.

Because of the large share of crimes in which information on alcohol use could not be ascertained, data on conjunctive combinations of alcohol use by offender and victim, such as the proportion of occurrences in which both had been drinking, are not presented here. These estimates would include a high proportion of cases where alcohol use for either participant was not known or recorded, to the point where the estimates could become quite misleading. For violent crimes in the community, I will therefore only report proportions of offenders and victims who were recorded as having been drinking, as well as the disjunctive combination of total alcohol involvement.

Patterns of Alcohol Involvement by Offenders and Victims

When the police recording of violent crime incidents is taken at its face value, the offenders had used alcohol in 31% of the incidents. For the victims this was true in 26% of the cases, and in 42% either one or both of the participants had been drinking ($n = 749$).[2] The latter figure is, of course, the standard measure of total alcohol involvement in methodologically parallel investigations from different parts of the world (see Chapter 2). Considering the high proportion of victims and offenders whose alcohol use was not known, it is perhaps remarkable that alcohol was recorded as being involved in 42% of violent crimes in the community (or 39% if we include victims under 15 and offenders under 12). It

2. Offenders under the age of 12 and victims under age 15 have been left out in calculating these proportions. If they are included, the total alcohol involvement was 39%, and offenders and victims had been drinking in 28% and 24% of the violent crimes, respectively.

may also be noted that this is very close to the estimate arrived at for homicides in the whole of Canada for the period 1961–1974, which was about 44% (Statistics Canada, 1976).

Gender-Related Patterns

We will later see that recorded violent crimes in the community showed a somewhat different picture of alcohol involvement from the sample of violence episodes covered in the survey. Still, the main patterns were similar. Contrary to survey findings, however, police-recorded violence in which women had been victimized had a higher degree of total alcohol involvement (46%) than crimes with male victims (39%), as shown in Table 6.2 (cf. Table 6.6, below). The rather high level of

TABLE 6.2. Alcohol Involvement in Violent Crimes as Related to Gender and Age of Offender and Victim

	Total alcohol involvement	Drinking by:	
		Offender	Victim
Total (n = 749)	42%	31%	26%
Gender of victim			
Male (n = 383)	39%	23%	29%
Female (n = 366)	46%	39%	23%
Gender of offender			
Male (n = 692)	43%	32%	27%
With male victim (n = 364)	39%	23%	30%
With female victim (n = 328)	48%	41%	23%
Female (n = 57)	30%	19%	19%
Age of victim			
Under 15 (n = 77)	5%	5%	0%
15–19 (n = 163)	29%	22%	19%
20–29 (n = 221)	44%	29%	30%
30–39 (n = 119)	46%	33%	31%
40–49 (n = 98)	53%	41%	28%
50 and over (n = 91)	47%	29%	34%
Age of offender			
Under 15 (n = 37)	0%	0%	0%
15–19 (n = 141)	26%	18%	14%
20–29 (n = 282)	39%	27%	25%
30–39 (n = 129)	45%	36%	26%
40–49 (n = 79)	61%	52%	35%
50 and over (n = 57)	46%	39%	18%

alcohol use by offenders of female victims (39%) is not entirely unexpected, considering the links between problem drinking and domestic violence reported in the literature. According to the police reports, male victims had consumed alcohol in a greater proportion of incidents than had their assailants. Here the discrepant proportions of offenders whose alcohol use was not known may have had some effect, though.

Another way in which the police data differ from the survey results is the small difference in the proportion of prior alcohol use by male and female victims (Table 6.2; cf. Table 6.6, below). The relatively high total alcohol involvement and alcohol use by the offenders in female victimizations may in part be an artifact of the closer relationship between offenders and victims in these cases, leading to more complete information on the offenders' drinking. However, the comparatively high proportion of alcohol consumption by female victims themselves is not as easily explained away. It is perhaps true in many communities that a subsegment of residents, which is too small to affect the findings from general population samples to any notable extent, is overrepresented in violence that comes to the attention of the police. This would give rise to different patterns of alcohol involvement than is the case in the general population. I have noted earlier that violent crimes tend to cluster among certain individuals and groups of individuals, and that it is also heavily concentrated among subsegments of alcohol abusers. This is generally true for both victims and offenders in violent crime.

Both the police census and the interview survey found that men were more likely to be victimized by strangers than were women. This may in part explain the low drinking prevalence among the victimizers of men in violent crime, since drinking by a person not known by the police (and the victim) would be less likely to have been noted on the occurrence sheet. This possibility is examined later with these violent crime data.

Alcohol use by both offenders and victims was much more common in the incidents in which the offenders were male (Table 6.2). The comparatively high proportion of alcohol use by the offenders (41%)—and, as a result, the high total alcohol involvement—in crimes with male offenders and female victims (48%), is noteworthy (Table 6.2) and is examined in some detail later in discussing the relationship between participants.

Age-Related Patterns

Drinking by the victims showed a fairly stable proportion of about 30% after the age of 20 (Table 6.2). As with victims, assailants in their 40s had the highest total alcohol involvement and also the highest level of their own drinking. The highest proportion of alcohol use was found among assailants in their 40s and their victims, contrary to the findings from the interview episodes (cf. Table 6.8 below). The public visibility of behavior in different segments of the population, and the *modus operandi* of the police in surveying and guarding the streets and neighborhoods, are significant factors in explaining these differences. It seems likely that violence occurring among heavily drinking individuals of low social status in almost any community comes to the attention of the police more readily than violence in other segments of society. On the other hand, the police and the public often take a looser view of violence that occurs in predominantly alcohol-abusing groups, especially if such groups are ecologically contained in "skid row" and similar areas, and do not enforce the law as strictly as in other, less notorious groups or areas. Community and police concern about the violence of this stratum is more acute if the violence is less restricted geographically and more visible to the general population. This probably makes it subject to considerable local, and to some extent temporal, variations.

The patterns of alcohol involvement in recorded violent crime probably also reflect the extent of heavy long-term alcohol use and alcoholism in the offenders more than does violence accessed through general population studies (especially if all respondents are represented by a maximum of one violent episode in the latter studies). Younger individuals who commit violent crimes and do not chronically abuse alcohol are gradually weeded out of community violence, whereas abusers of alcohol have a continued high risk of participating in violent encounters into their later years. In other words, nonabusers of alcohol leave their violent "careers" with rising age, while abusers are more likely to persist in violent behavior patterns. As an outcome of these joint processes, the incidence of violent crime decreases with age, whereas the alcohol involvement in these crimes may well increase. This is indicated by the high proportions of offenders aged 40 and over who had been drinking prior to violence (Table 6.2).

It is also noteworthy that drinking by the victims in violent crime showed a rather steady increase between the ages of 15 and 19, where alcohol involvement (and perhaps drinking patterns) seemed to stabilize. The percentages of drinking victims for these ages were as follows, starting with the 15-year-olds: 12%, 11%, 15%, 27% and 28%. The corresponding proportions of offenders who had been drinking were 0%, 19%, 13%, 29%, and 19%. The base numbers were small, ranging between 26 and 40 for victims and 15 and 42 for offenders, but the age pattern was still clear.

Location-Related Patterns

The main difference between violent episodes accessed through the interview study and the ones that came to the attention of the community police was the relatively high relation to alcohol use of the violent crimes that occurred in a private home (Table 6.3; cf. Table 6.8, below). Returning to Table 6.1 makes it evident that this finding would persist even if we were only to consider the violence in which the assailant's identity was definitely known. Conceivably, it is in part a reflection of the disproportionate effort that the police have to expend on families in which one or more adults have serious problems related to alcohol use.

The relatively low level of alcohol involvement in violent crimes committed in public drinking places is another sign of the minimum nature of the alcohol use estimates derived from the police census data (cf. the high level of alcohol involvement in the interview survey, discussed below). Victims in this setting were recorded with a higher

TABLE 6.3. Alcohol Involvement in Violent Crimes as Related to Location of Incident, Number of Participants, and the Relationship between Victim and (Main) Offender

	Total alcohol involvement	Drinking by:	
		Offender	Victim
Total (n = 749)	42%	31%	26%
Location			
Private home (n = 336)	44%	39%	22%
Work or school (n = 13)	8%	8%	0%
Public drinking place (n = 77)	65%	40%	52%
Street or park (n = 225)	43%	23%	30%
Hotel or motel (n = 20)	55%	35%	55%
Other location (n = 92)	17%	8%	11%
Number of participants			
One offender (n = 626)	42%	32%	24%
More than one offender (n = 139)	47%	23%	36%
One victim (n = 702)	41%	29%	26%
More than one victim (n = 61)	57%	46%	36%
Relationship			
Spouse or common-law partner (n = 160)	47%	43%	16%
Other family member (n = 47)	36%	23%	21%
Acquaintance or friend (n = 305)	40%	33%	34%
Stranger (n = 178)	43%	29%	28%
Relationship unknown (n = 78)	49%	24%	32%

level of alcohol use (52%) than were offenders (40%). It is noteworthy that this was also the case for only victims and offenders whose exact birth dates were recorded (61% and 50%, respectively; from Table 6.1). The category "other locations" includes arenas and stadiums, stores, shopping malls, restaurants not licensed to serve alcohol, public service areas or offices (welfare office, lawyer's office, etc.), buses, cars, and so forth. The mundane, "daily business" character of these areas no doubt explains much of the absence of alcohol. Although the "other location" category in Table 6.1 includes some additional locations compared to the classification in Table 6.3 (with a total n of 145, compared to 92 in the latter table), it is evident that even offenders whose identity was known had been drinking less often than similar offenders in the "other location" category.

Other Patterns

There was practically no difference in alcohol involvement between events in which there was more than one offender and those in which there was only one offender (Table 6.3). (The coders were instructed to record the characteristics of the most active assailant, and if this was not possible, to randomly select one of the offenders for inclusion in the sample and the recording of alcohol use.) Contrary to violence episodes from the interviews (cf. Table 6.9 below), the offender was reported as having been drinking less often when there was more than one offender (23% vs. 32%; $\chi^2 = 4.17$, $df = 1$, $p < .05$). Viewed from the same type of stereotyped descriptive hypothesis, the fact that more victims in multiple-offender violent crimes (36%) were recorded as having consumed alcohol than were offenders (23%) is also unexpected ($\chi^2 = 5.62$, $df = 1$, $p < .02$). Perhaps some of these incidents were robberies or robbery attempts perpetrated by groups of youths.

In the case of multiple victims, there was a higher likelihood of alcohol consumption by the (designated) victim (36% vs. 26%). The overall alcohol involvement was also significantly higher (57%) when there were multiple victims ($\chi^2 = 5.15$, $df = 1$, $p < .05$) than with single victims (41%), and so was drinking by the (designated) offender (46% vs. 29%; $\chi^2 = 6.63$, $df = 1$, $p < .02$).

Total alcohol involvement did not differ very much between different relationships in the violent crimes of the community (Table 6.3). The greatest discrepancy in the share of drinking offenders and drinking victims was found in marital violence. There was a difference of 27 percentage points between these prevalence figures, whereas these differed by only 2 to 8 percentage points in the other types of relationships. Obviously, the family violence in which the community police must become involved is a rather one-sided affair in terms of alcohol use.

Concluding Comments

By way of summary, it can be said that this study, like many other North American studies that have used police records as sources of data, has probably underestimated the involvement of alcohol in serious violent behavior. Still, fully 42% of the violent crimes that occurred in the study community were noted by the police to be alcohol-related, and it is quite possible—considering the suspiciously low level of registered alcohol use in the violence occurring in public drinking places—that the true figure of total alcohol involvement could well reach 55–60%.

The discrepancies in the sampling of violent crime episodes and the most recent episodes of victimization reported in the interview survey have already been discussed. In moving to a consideration of alcohol involvement in the latter episodes, I should first of all note that this is probably the first time that the alcohol involvement in violence episodes have been studied by direct sampling within a general population. Practically no systematic knowledge is available on the role that alcohol plays in "everyday" violence (i.e., violence that is not necessarily recorded by legal authorities, health or social agencies, health professionals, etc., and that is free of the self-selection biases inherent in visits to the latter two types of sources and in reporting patterns to the police).

ALCOHOL INVOLVEMENT IN VIOLENCE REPORTED IN INTERVIEWS

Fifteen percent of the violent situations that were tapped through the interviews had led to the police's "being involved," and 6% had led to formal charges' being laid (see questions 21 and 22 in Appendix B). This should be compared to the 100% police attention of the violent crime incidents just discussed. In addition, it is very likely that the police never recorded a proportion of these 15% even though they were made aware that they had taken place. (In this context, it is relevant that only 4% of incidents of physical violence were recorded by police, according to the earlier estimate based on violent incidents that occurred during a 12-month period.) Thus a maximum of 15% of interview study episodes were such that they would have been available in any samples drawn from police census material, and 6% would have been included in any study based on court records. (If samples had been taken from visits to hospitals or health professionals for medical care, 11% of the violence episodes from the survey would have been available for inclusion; see Chapter 8. An unknown, but probably much lower, proportion would have been available for emergency room studies.) We are thus dealing with a very different sampling universe when we study the violence reported by respondents in the interviews carried out in the study community. Despite the relatively awkward sampling perspective that the interview data introduce, they are still probably much more representative of the types of violence occurring among the general public in daily life than are the samples from police or health care sources. Even from this narrow perspective, a study of such episodes has value. It should be evident from the discussion below that a great many questions can be asked in a study of this kind that are not possible in studies using the traditional sources of data.

Drinking by Assailants versus Victims

Alcohol had been used by one or both participants in 53.6% of the sampled episodes of physical violence ($n = 412$). (There were 37 missing values; 3 respondents did not remember whether they had themselves been drinking, and 34 respondents did not know or remember whether their assailants had been drinking.) This is very close to the modal figure reported in North American studies of official records of violent crime (mostly homicides—see reviews by Pernanen, 1976, and Roizen & Schneberk, 1977). Both the respondent and his/her assailant had been drinking in 27.1% of these situations; in 23.8%, only the assailant had consumed alcohol; and the respondent was the sole drinker in only 2.7% of the violent episodes.

By adding up the relevant categories, we find that the assailant had been drinking in just over half (51%) of the occasions when violence occurred. The respondent had been drinking in 30% of these occasions. Obviously, alcohol use was very much part of the violence experienced by city residents. Considering the wide spread of these occasions over time, and to some extent also the geographical spread, it is of interest to note that the total alcohol involvement in the violence that had occurred within the city limits during the last 8 years was 60% ($n = 219$), and that the alcohol use combinations did not differ much from the ones found in the total sample of violent episodes (with only the respondent drinking in 2%, only the assailant in 26%, and both participants in 29% of the incidents).

The proportion of episodes in which only the respondent/victim had been drinking was extremely low, compared to the proportion in which only the assailant had consumed alcohol. There are several possible explanations for this. If we assume that there is a greater probability of a physical attack by a person who is under the influence of alcohol and a low probability of retaliation by a sober victim, we would expect more attackers (assailants) than targets of attack (victims, and in the present methodology, respondents) to be intoxicated. The subset of violent incidents accessed by selecting the most recent occasion in which a respondent was the *victim* of violent acts would under such circumstances not include many incidents in which only the respondent himself/herself had been drinking and aggressed physically against another person, since there would be victimization of the attacker/respondent (and the event would consequently be included in the sample of violent events) only if there was some physical resistance or retaliation by the sober adversary. Occasions on which only one person acted in a violent manner were included in this interview survey only if the victim did not retaliate, because of the selection procedure of the survey (and other typical victimization surveys). The inclusion in the sample of relatively few cases in which only a victimized respondent had been drinking would in that case be due to the fact that his/her sober antagonist had attacked, retaliated, or put up active physical resistance in very few cases. Selective mechanisms of this nature do not exist in direct samples of incidents, such as the violent crime occurrences found in police records, but are built into samples of the general population in which (1) participants report on events that (2) are not weighted by the probability of an individual's being involved in violence.

If this factor alone were to account for the difference between the proportions of events in which the antagonist alone and the respondent alone had been drinking, we could—on the basis of these "alone-drinking" figures and some *ceteris paribus* assumptions—calculate the likelihood of retaliation by a sober person who had initially been subjected to violence by a person who had consumed alcohol. The ratio between the incidence of events in which the antagonist alone had been drinking and the ones in which the respondent alone had been drinking was $23.8 \div 2.7 = 8.8$. Thus, the probability of a sober person's retaliating when subjected to some violent act by a person who had been drinking was only about 1 in 10. However, we have to remember again that we are not dealing with an incidence sample of episodes, and in order for this reasoning to hold true we have to assume that the two-stage systematic sample reflects essential features of a simple random sample of violent episodes.

Several other alternative or supplementary explanations for the discrepancy between the antagonist and the respondent as the lone drinker in violence suggest themselves. One of these is that assaults occurring in connection with drinking only by the respondent show a low prevalence because drunken aggression is concentrated among relatively few individuals who become assaultive while under the influence of alcohol. The few "mean drunks" who happened to be included in the present sample of respondents were only represented by one incident in which they had been drinking (the "drinking by the respondent" category) if the other persons involved also acted in some violent manner toward these respondents (who thus became victimized); however, these respondents would potentially appear as (drinking) antagonists in several aggressive incidents reported by community residents. (In the illustration given near the end of Chapter 5, Sue would qualify as such a person; in the course of a few minutes, she physically attacked at least four male patrons in the tavern.) Several studies in North America and Europe have shown that there is an overrepresentation in violent crime of individuals who belong to marginal subgroups and have a previous record of violent crimes and other types of crime (e.g., Macdonald, 1967; McClintock, 1963; Wikström, 1985; Wolfgang, 1958). The violence perpetrated by these individuals is mainly of an ingroup nature, but also includes conflicts with members of more typical segments of the general public. In addition, there exist among alcoholics subgroups that have been designated *inter alia* as "violent," "dangerous," "assaultive," or "belligerent" (e.g., Berglund & Tunving, 1985; Hagnell, Nyman, & Tunving, 1973; Löberg, 1983; Renson, Adams, & Tinklenberg, 1978; Schuckit & Russell, 1984). On the basis of this explanatory possibility, one would expect violence in cases where the assailant was a total stranger to have a relatively great proportion of alcohol involvement.

A related possible explanation of the discrepancy arising out of such a skewed distribution of alcohol-related aggression is that these assaultive drinkers may fall outside the sampling frame of a study such as the present one, because they live in places that are difficult to enumerate or find. They may also be more likely to end up as cases of attrition because they do not have a telephone, are more likely not to be at home, change their place of residence frequently, are more likely to refuse, or are in a condition that does not allow them to be interviewed. Consequently, this category of persons would be more likely to show up in the survey sample of violence episodes as drinking assailants than as drinking respondents. A combination of these types of factors probably explains a major part of the low prevalence of physical victimizations in which only the respondent had been drinking.

At the very least, it can be said that the proportions of alcohol involvement in the present interview survey are incompatible at their face value with the assumption that a drinking and a nondrinking person would have equal probabilities of attacking or retaliating physically in response to an attack. The interpretations offered above, of course, rest entirely on differential probabilities in this regard.[3] In order to assess these interpretations and their underlying assumptions properly, we would, at a minimum, need information on the extent to which respondents in the survey retaliated physically in some way or even initiated the physical violence. Such information was not obtained. Some consolation is provided by the fact that cumulative research efforts thrive on such hindsights.

Amounts of Alcohol Consumed

Out of the 206 violence episodes in which the opponent was judged to have been drinking, he/she was assessed by the respondent to have been "drunk" in 68% of these. This accounted for 32% of all violence. There did not seem to be any relationship between drinking by the victim and the likelihood that he/she would judge the assailant to be drunk. The respondent was drinking in about 47% of the incidents in which the antagonist was judged to be drunk ($n = 140$), and 53% of the events in which he/she was drinking but not drunk ($n = 66$). Amounts of alcohol consumed by the victim did not show any relationship to assessed drunkenness of the antagonist. This defining characteristic of a "drunken brawl" therefore did not seem to typify the violence in which both adversaries had been drinking. At face value, this can be interpreted as indicating that the threshold to violence is passed at lower levels of consumption (i.e., if at least one of the drinking participants is intoxicated), and that no increase in this probability occurs if *both* have been drinking excessively. It may also indicate that other determinants present in the situation are decisive, independently of the joint level of alcohol use.

On the other hand, when we look at the mean amounts of alcohol consumed (thereby letting high amounts consumed prior to violence have their full impact), a slight tendency toward a positive relationship between levels of drinking of the adversaries is discernible. In incidents of physical violence where the other person was judged to have been drunk, the respondent had consumed a mean of 9.6 cl of absolute alcohol ($n = 56$), the equivalent of about five and a half bottles of Canadian beer or the same number of 1½-ounce drinks of liquor. When the antagonist

3. We may obtain still another (partial) explanation for this pattern by assuming that there was selection bias in the *second* stage of sampling the violent episodes. Such a bias would have come about, for example, if respondents had been less willing to report or able to recall episodes of violence in which they had been drinking, or had tended not to reveal their own alcohol use in the events reported.

was not assessed as having been drunk, this mean was 8.1 cl ($n = 30$). Because of the very large range, the skewed distribution of these amounts, and the small base numbers, the difference between these means was not even close to acceptable levels of statistical significance.

The distribution of amounts consumed by respondents who had been drinking in the most recent violent episode is shown in Table 6.4. The categorization of volumes consumed has been made to coincide with common consumption units. The interval of 1.7 cl equals the alcohol content of a bottle of Canadian beer, a shot of 1½ ounces of distilled spirits, or about 5 ounces of table wine. For comparison, the table also includes the distribution of consumption in three types of recent drinking events that were asked about in the survey (see questions 63, 78, and 92 in Appendix B).

Overall, the respondents who reported drinking prior to the violent episode had consumed an average of 9.2 cl of 100% alcohol, with a median value at 6.7 cl ($n = 113$). This mean was about double the mean consumption of all nonabstaining respondents at their most recent drinking occasion in a private home or in a public drinking place (Table 6.4). It was about equal to the mean amount consumed by these respondents at the occasion during the 30 days preceding the interview when

TABLE 6.4. Amounts of Alcohol Consumed by Victims in the Most Recent Episodes of Physical Violence, by City Residents in Their Most Recent Episodes of Alcohol Use in a Private Home and a Public Drinking Place, and by City Residents on the Occasion of Maximum Consumption during the Last 30 days (in Centiliters of 100% Alcohol)

		Consumption at most recent drinking occasion		
Amount	Victims' consumption prior to violence ($n = 127$)	In a private home ($n = 780$)	In a public place ($n = 708$)	When maximum consumed[a] ($n = 783$)
0.1–1.7 cl	8%	41%	22%	12%
1.8–3.4 cl	14%	28%	27%	20%
3.5–6.8 cl	30%	19%	32%	28%
6.9–10.2 cl	22%	6%	11%	15%
10.3–13.6 cl	9%	3%	6%	10%
13.7–17.0 cl	4%	2%	1%	4%
17.1 cl and over	13%	1%	2%	11%

Note. Mean amounts of 100% alcohol consumed: victims, 9.2 cl; most recent occasion at home, 3.5 cl; most recent occasion in public drinking place, 5.0 cl; maximum, 8.3 cl. Median amounts of 100% alcohol consumed: victims, 6.7 cl; most recent occasion at home, 2.2 cl; most recent occasion at public drinking place, 3.9 cl; maximum, 5.8 cl. Note that percentages in some columns may not total 100% because of rounding.
[a]For 71 infrequent drinkers (9.1% of all alcohol users), a reference period of 12 months was used.

they consumed more alcohol than on any other occasion (for infrequently drinking respondents, who constituted 9.1% of the total sample, a reference period of 12 months was used). The mean of 9.2 cl corresponds to about 8 ounces of distilled spirits. The highest amount consumed by any respondent/victim prior to violence was 47 cl, the equivalent of about 42 ounces of distilled spirits.

The proportion of events in which relatively large amounts of alcohol were consumed by the respondents was considerably greater in violence episodes than on typical alcohol use occasions. However, the compositions of these samples differed considerably; for example, there were more men (especially young men) in the violence sample. We can nevertheless draw the superficial descriptive conclusion that occasions on which people drink more than average are more likely to be related to physical violence. This statement does not yet suggest anything about the causal pathways and alcohol's role in these; nor does it suggest that other factors are not of causal significance.

A partial test of whether drinking by a person later victimized in violence was atypically high could be accomplished through comparing the consumption in violence episodes and typical drinking occasions by holding constant the most central demographic characteristics of respondents/victims. With the cautionary note that the reports of consumption in drinking situations reflected drinking patterns at the time of the survey, whereas consumption reported for violence episodes pertained to a period on the average much further removed in time, we can also compare the victims' consumption prior to violence with their regular drinking episode consumption. This has been done in Table 6.5. In order to examine the effect of a decrease in temporal discrepancy between the most recent violence episodes and the most recent drinking occasions, I have also included the corresponding results for individuals whose events of violence occurred within 8 years of the interview date and within city limits.

First of all, there were no differences of any consequence in the victims' mean or median consumption between the total samples of violence episodes and those that had occurred in the city within the last 8 years prior to the interview. The more substantive question—whether the consumption reported by the victims in the violence events differed from their typical or maximum consumption—can be approached by comparing the means and medians of the first row with the figures for the three types of drinking episodes in the next three rows. It is evident that the amounts from the violence situations were considerably greater than the amounts drunk by the same persons on their last drinking occasions in a private home and in a public drinking establishment. However, they were also much below the maximum amounts consumed.

TABLE 6.5. Median and Mean Amounts of Alcohol Consumed by Victims of Physical Violence, and Median and Mean Amounts of Alcohol Consumed by the *Same* Respondents on the Most Recent Drinking Occasions in a Private Home and a Public Drinking Place, and on the Occasion of Maximum Consumption (in Centiliters of 100% Alcohol)

	Mean		Median	
Type of drinking occasion	All	In community within 8 years	All	In community within 8 years
Violence episode (n's = 127/71)[a]	9.2	9.0	6.7	6.7
Most recent drinking occasion:				
In a home (n's = 127/71)[a]	5.1	5.2	3.4	3.4
In a public drinking place (n's = 124/70)[a]	6.8	6.8	5.1	5.6
At maximum consumption (n's = 126/70)[a]	13.4	14.0	10.1	11.2

[a]The first n is the total sample size for victimization events in which the victim had been drinking prior to violence; the second n is the sample size for the subsample of events in the community in the eight years preceding the interview.

One tentative conclusion to be drawn from these findings is that high alcohol consumption levels by themselves do not determine involvement in violence, since (1) the maximum consumption levels were well above the consumption levels in the violence events; (2) very few of these occasions of maximum alcohol consumption led to angry arousal; and (3) even fewer resulted in open aggression and physical violence.[4] Therefore, other factors have to be present in addition to sufficient levels of alcohol use for physical violence to ensue in human interaction. However, another conclusion from these findings is that at victimization the victim seems to have consumed more alcohol than he/she usually does.

It can also be tentatively concluded that victimization cannot be attributed completely to deviant drinking habits of the victims. On the other hand, a comparison between the average amounts in Tables 6.4 and 6.5 shows that victims of aggression consumed more on fairly typical occasions than drinkers in the general population. For instance, the median and mean levels of consumption in a public drinking establishment for the drinkers in the total interview sample were 3.9 cl and 5.0 cl, respectively (see first footnote to Table 6.4). Among individuals who had been drinking when last subjected to violence, the median and mean were 5.1 cl and 6.8 cl, respectively (see Table 6.5).

4. Patterns of angry arousal and behavior linked to it will be reported in the upcoming monograph described in Chapter 1, footnote 1.

Patterns of Alcohol Involvement by Assailants and Victims

Gender-Related Patterns

It has been stated earlier that out of the 451 violent incidents reported on by the respondents, 232 or 51% occurred between men, and 38 or 8% between women. In addition, 144 women (32%) had a male assailant, and 36 men (8%) had a female assailant.

Women who were victimized reported a lower proportion of assailants who had been drinking (45%) than did male victims (54%; Table 6.6). On these occasions, female victims had themselves also been drinking to a much lesser extent than had male victims. The total alcohol involvement was 59% in incidents in which men reported being victimized and 47% in incidents where the victims were women. Episodes in which only the victims had been drinking were consistently low in all the different subgroups of the population, ranging between 0% and 4%. They have been left out of Table 6.6 and the other alcohol involvement tables for the sake of easier reviewing of the results.

The assailant was deemed by female victims to have been "drunk" in 28% of the incidents, compared to 34% of the victimizations of men. There was no difference in the proportion of drunk assailants out of the

TABLE 6.6. Alcohol Use by the Assailant and Victim Prior to the Most Recent Episode of Physical Violence, as Related to the Gender of the Victim and Assailant

	Total alcohol involvement	Drinking by: Assailant	Victim	Both	*Only* assailant
Total sample (n's = 418/451)[a]	54%	51%	30%	26%	22%
Male victim (n's = 248/269)[a]	59%	54%	37%	33%	18%
Female victim (n's = 172/182)[a]	47%	45%	18%	16%	29%
Male assailant (n's = 345/366)[a]	58%	56%	31%	28%	26%
With male victim (n's = 209/226)[a]	62%	59%	40%	37%	20%
With female victim (n's = 136/143)[a]	53%	51%	18%	15%	35%
Female assailant (n's = 71/73)[a]	27%	21%	21%	15%	4%

[a]See text for an explanation of the double base figures.

events in which the assailant had been drinking (63% for assailants of male victims and 64% for assailants of female victims). At its surface value, this finding tends to disconfirm any hypothesis that higher thresholds of alcohol use or BACs are necessary for physical aggression against a woman as compared to physical aggression against a man. At least, it seems safe to conclude that other determining factors outweigh any such tendencies if they exist.

A Note on Estimates of Alcohol Involvement

Before the discussion advances any further, the double base figures shown in Table 6.6 and some subsequent tables need to be explained, as well as the labels attached to the five columns. The base figures vary for the different estimates of alcohol involvement. Total alcohol involvement in an episode (i.e., the percentage of episodes in which at least one of the adversaries had been drinking) could be ascertained even if it was not known whether the assailant had been drinking, as long as it was known that the respondent/victim had been drinking. The same, of course, was true of the share of episodes in which the respondent had been drinking (the "Drinking by victim" column in the tables) and those in which the assailant had been drinking (the "Drinking by assailant" column); these episodes could be categorized regardless of whether the other person's drinking was known or not. I illustrate the point with the "Drinking by victim'" column in Table 6.6. This column includes (1) events in which both adversaries had been drinking; (2) events in which only the respondent had been drinking; and (3) events in which the respondent had been drinking, but it was not known whether the assailant had been drinking. In order for an event to be classified as one in which both the assailant and the victim had been drinking, on the other hand, the cases in which the assailant's drinking was not known have had to be considered as missing values, even if it was known that the respondent had been drinking. Thus the bases of the estimates are generally smaller. The two different base figures shown in the tables on alcohol involvement refer to these two alternative bases. The higher figure is the base for the estimates of the proportions of "Drinking by assailant," "Drinking by victim," and the total alcohol involvement of the episodes. The lower figure is the base for the estimates of the proportion of incidents in which both participants and only the assailant had been drinking—that is, incidents for the classification of which information was needed about the drinking of both adversaries. This type of utilization of the data has led to some (on the whole insignificant) discrepancies in these tables. These emerge, for instance, when the totals of the percentages for "Drinking by both," "Drinking by only assailant," and the percentage of episodes in which only the victim had been drinking (not shown in tables) do not tally with the figure for total alcohol involvement. (The maximum difference is 4 percentage points.)

At the right in Table 6.6 and other alcohol involvement tables are the two least problematic columns. These indicate the percentage of violence episodes prior to which *only* the assailant (but not the victim) had been drinking, and the percentage of episodes prior to which both victim and assailant had consumed alcohol. The "Drinking by victim" column includes the incidents where both adversaries had been drinking ("Drinking by both"), as well as the incidents where only the victim had done so (as mentioned earlier, this is not shown separately because of its low share—an average of 2%). The "Drinking by assailant" column includes the proportion of incidents in which both participants had been drinking and the proportion in which only the assailant had been drinking. In principle, the percentages of the two columns on the right should add up to the percentage in this column, but they do not because of the maximum utilization of the data with shifting bases (in addition to the effect of some rounding discrepancies). Finally, as I have stated earlier, the percentages in the "Total alcohol involvement" column comprise incidents in which both had been drinking, the assailant only had been drinking, and the victim only had been drinking.

In presenting the findings, I continue to refer to the respondent as "the victim," in keeping with the practice of victimization surveys. As already mentioned, this does not imply that "the assailant" invariably started the conflict or a physical altercation, or that the respondent was the only one who sustained injuries or had valid reason for complaining to the authorities. However, this was probably the case in a majority of the episodes accessed through interviews with community residents.

Further Gender-Related Patterns

Now let us return to the examination of substantive findings. Table 6.7 shows the mean consumption of all male and female respondents (both those who had been and those who had not been victimized through violence since the age of 15) who had consumed alcohol at least once in a private home and in a drinking establishment during the 12 months preceding the interview. The mean consumption in the drinking situation when respondents consumed more alcohol than on any other occasion during the last 30 days (or 12 months for infrequent drinkers) is also shown in the table. The amounts consumed by men and women on the occasions when they were victimized (9.9 cl and 6.2 cl, respectively) were considerably higher than the mean levels of consumption during the most recent drinking episodes in a home or in a public drinking place. The amounts preceding the violent episodes were

TABLE 6.7. Mean Amounts of Alcohol Consumed by Men and Women in the Most Recent Drinking Occasions in a Private Home and a Public Drinking Place, and on the Occasion of Maximum Consumption (in Centiliters of 100% Alcohol)

	Men ($n = 456$)	Women ($n = 356$)	Total ($n = 812$)
In a private home	4.3	2.5	3.5
In a public drinking place	6.0	3.8	5.0
Maximum consumption	10.7	5.3	8.3

much closer to the maximum amounts consumed on one occasion for both genders; they were somewhat lower for men, but higher for women.

Male assailants had been drinking in 56% of the community residents' most recent violent victimizations (Table 6.6). The corresponding percentage for women as assailants, 21%, was much lower. The respondents judged male antagonists to have been "drunk" in 36% of the episodes, whereas female antagonists were so judged in 15% of the incidents. The total alcohol involvement for episodes with male victimizers was 58%, compared to 27% when a woman had acted violently toward the respondent.

Violence involving only men as participants had the highest total alcohol involvement of all gender combinations, 62% (Table 6.6). This resulted in large measure from the relatively great number of incidents in which both the respondent and his antagonist had been drinking. Episodes in which the assailant was male and the victimized respondent was a woman had an alcohol involvement figure of 53%. These alcohol-related cases mainly consisted of events in which only the assailant (i.e., the male) had been drinking.

Age-Related Patterns

The age distribution of the victimized respondents and their assailants at the time of the most recent violence has been discussed in Chapter 5. For both men and women, there was a solid concentration among young age groups. With regard to the presence of alcohol, victims in their 20s had been drinking in 41% of their encounters with violence, more often than any other age group (Table 6.8). Among the youngest of the four age groups, those aged between 15 and 19 at the time of violence, only 17% had been drinking prior to becoming victims. With the exception of the youngest respondents, the rates of total alcohol involvement were fairly similar in the different age groups, despite the peak of drinking by victims in their 20s. With increasing age in the adult years, total alcohol use proportions stayed high through an increase in the share of incidents in which only the antagonist had been drinking. There was a corresponding decline in the proportion of events in which both actors had been drinking. "Drunken brawls," as noted earlier, seem to be a phenomenon of young adulthood. The increase with age in proportions of events in which only the antagonist had been drinking shows the increasing one-sidedness of the role of alcohol in violence with increasing age. It is probably related to the greater tendency of women to have experienced their most recent victimization at a relatively late age.

Mean amounts of alcohol consumed by the respondents who had been drinking when last subjected to violent acts did not differ much between age groups, in the face of low base numbers and large variances. They varied between 7.9 cl in the youngest age group and 9.6 cl in the two middle categories. By comparison, the highest amounts on all three types of drinking occasions were consumed by men and women in their

TABLE 6.8. Alcohol Use by the Assailant and Victim Prior to the Most Recent Episode of Physical Violence, as Related to the Age of the Victim and Assailant at the Time of the Episode and to the Location of the Episode

	Total alcohol involvement	Drinking by:			
		Assailant	Victim	Both	*Only* assailant
Total sample (*n*'s = 418/451)	54%	51%	30%	26%	22%
Age of victim					
Under 20 (*n*'s = 101/105)	28%	25%	17%	14%	10%
20–29 (*n*'s = 156/171)	64%	62%	41%	38%	21%
30–39 (*n*'s = 72/77)	57%	54%	27%	25%	28%
40 and over (*n*'s = 75/82)	65%	61%	27%	23%	37%
Age of assailant					
Under 20 (*n*'s = 97/103)	26%	23%	14%	11%	11%
20–29 (*n*'s = 161/177)	68%	65%	41%	37%	25%
30–39 (*n*'s = 71/75)	58%	54%	37%	32%	21%
40 and over (*n*'s = 84/90)	50%	48%	18%	17%	31%
Location of violence					
Victim's home (*n*'s = 149/155)	39%	36%	15%	12%	24%
Other home (*n*'s = 46/47)	70%	66%	46%	40%	23%
Work or school (*n*'s = 64/68)	25%	23%	8%	6%	17%
Public drinking place (*n*'s = 66/70)	99%	97%	79%	77%	16%
Street or park (*n*'s = 50/61)	48%	44%	13%	9%	34%
Other location (*n*'s = 34/39)	56%	53%	36%	32%	18%

20s. In the maximum consumption episode, men of this age had drunk 14.5 cl ($n = 117$) and women 7.0 cl ($n = 110$) of absolute alcohol, for a total mean of 10.9 cl (i.e., somewhat more than the 9.6 cl when last victimized).

Drinking by participants in violence as related to the age of the assailant showed patterns similar to those related to the age of the victim (Table 6.8). (This should come as no great surprise, since we have seen that the ages of participants in violent events tended to be similar.) Assailants in their 20s were most likely to have been drinking prior to the violence; almost two-thirds had done so. Those aged over 30 had rates of about 50%, and the youngest age group a very low rate, 23%.

The total alcohol involvement in incidents with assailants in their 20s was high, 68% (Table 6.8). The rates were also high in the other two adult age groups, 58% for assailants in their 30s and 50% for those in their 40s and older. (These results follow the relative order of drinking frequency by age; results not shown.) Violent incidents in which the assailant was between 15 and 19 years of age had a total alcohol involvement of only 26%.

According to the victims' assessment, 41% of the assailants in their 20s were "drunk" ($n = 161$); those in their 30s were judged to be in a drunken state in 37% of the violent incidents ($n = 71$). The youngest assailants, those aged under 20, had the lowest rate of assessed drunkenness in violence, 17% ($n = 97$). The oldest assailants (aged 40 and over) were "drunk" in 33% of the episodes ($n = 84$).

Location-Related Patterns

Men and women differed in the locations where they had experienced violence (figures not shown in tables). Fully 60% of the last violent encounters of women had occurred in the home; for men, the share was only 17%. One-fourth of male victimizations in violent incidents had taken place in a licensed drinking establishment; among women, this share was only 5%. We have seen earlier that, besides men and women, young, middle-aged, and older persons also differed in the extent to which they participated in aggression in homes, street or parks, taverns, and other locations. We might also expect different rates of alcohol involvement in the different locations of episodes, and thus among these groups of people, purely on the basis of the variations in locations where the violence occurred (and vice versa).

It stands to reason that the highest alcohol involvement figures would be found in the violence occurring in taverns and bars. In the survey, the total involvement of alcohol in physically violent episodes located in these establishments was 99% (i.e., the respondent, the antagonist, or both had been drinking in all cases but one; Table 6.8). The respondent/victim had not been drinking in about one-fifth of these incidents, whereas the assailant had consumed alcohol in almost all such events. Several of the nondrinking victims in taverns and bars were working as waiters, bartenders, or bouncers at the time. Employees of establishments licensed to serve alcohol are one of the occupational groups at high risk of involvement in aggressive encounters (e.g., Kraus, 1987). Other such groups are police officers and security guards (Hales, Seligman, Newman, & Timbrook, 1988; Kraus, 1987), bus and taxi drivers (Davis, 1987; Dietz & Baker, 1987), and emergency room personnel (Morgan & Steedman, 1986—with 70% of these assaultive individuals ($n = 109$), mostly patients, being intoxicated). A recent study of workplace homicides in Ontario between 1975 and 1985 ($n = 84$) found that policemen, gas station attendants, security guards, taxidrivers, and employees of jewelery stores, restaurants, and taverns had the highest risk of death by homicide (Liss & Craig, 1990). A fairly typical incident of aggressive conflict involving a tavern employee is the following, which was documented by one of the present study's observers in a city tavern.

> The setting was a typical downtown tavern with mainly working-class patronage, moderately high in aggressive incidents. One of the patrons being observed was "Grease," a man in his 30s. He was drunk and loud, and offended someone with his language. He was asked by the bartender to correct himself and apologize. Grease questioned the bartender's authority to make him retract what he had said and to make him apologize, and started to threaten the bartender with physical violence. The bartender replied, "You scare me. I'm terrified." At that point Grease was already walking toward the exit. At the door he turned around, looked at the bartender, and said, "Come on outside and I'll show you how fucking terrified you are." He then left the establishment.

At other times there were attempts at hurting tavern employees or actual subjections to violence. These were also reflected in several accounts from the interviews with city residents. In one such case, the respondent was about 20 years old at the time of the incident: "I was working at the bar and these two guys started a fight. We kind of helped them out the door, and they returned right away with baseball bats." However, physical violence did not come about: "We just locked the front doors and then just ignored them." In another case, the respondent (a plumber by occupation) had been working as a bartender in a local tavern. He had not been drinking at the time of his most recent victimization through physical violence. The assailant was a man in his 20s who was judged by the respondent to be drunk: "This man was barred from coming back to the hotel, and he was in when I came on shift. I asked him to leave, and he hit me with a beer bottle."

The presence of alcohol was also relatively high in a home other than the respondent's own (70%). Probably much of this violence occurred at parties. There was alcohol present in 39% of violence in the respondent's own home. The lowest prevalence of alcohol in any location was in the workplace or school of the respondent. Still, even here the total share of the presence of alcohol was as high as 25%.

Major differences between locations surfaced in the extent to which, on the one hand, both participants had been drinking and, on the other hand, the assailant only had been. In a street or park, there was a higher likelihood than in any other location that violence would occur between a sober respondent and an adversary who had been drinking. Somebody else's home and the miscellaneous "other location" category (summer cottage, hotel or motel, etc.) contained a fairly high proportion of events in which both adversaries had been drinking. Joint drinking situations naturally dominated in tavern and bar violence.

The results pertaining to the location of violence in effect show two distinct types of settings. In incidents occurring in a street or park, at work or school, and in the home of the victim, the proportion of alcohol-involved incidents in which only the assailant had been drinking was between 60% and 70%. In other private homes, public drinking establishments, and miscellaneous other settings, this proportion was about 20–30%.

The amounts consumed by the victims prior to violence varied widely; with the problematically low base figures in a detailed location breakdown, any generalizations would be ill advised. Tavern and bar incidents, however, had a large enough base ($n = 55$) to deserve cautious mention; in these, the respondent/victim had consumed a mean of 9.5 cl of 100% alcohol, which does not differ much from the overall mean of 9.2 cl. This can also be compared to a mean of 5.0 cl consumed by all respondents at their last drinking occasion in a licensed establishment.

Other Patterns

I have noted earlier that *more than one person* physically attacked the victim in 15% of violent events reported in the interviews with community residents. This was true for 20% of victimized men and 7% of female victims. In all probability, this difference again largely reflects the much greater share of domestic violence among women and the greater likelihood that men will be victimized outside the home, particularly in connection with tavern and bar drinking. Facing more than one antagonist implies a somewhat higher presence of alcohol use. The total alcohol involvement in events with one antagonist was 52%, and for events with more than one assailant it was 61% (Table 6.9). (The difference was not statistically significant.) This excess is accounted for by the greater proportion of events in which both principal participants had been drinking (the reader is reminded that in the case of multiple assailants, the respondent was asked to describe the one who was most active in victimizing him/her). It is no doubt a partial reflection of the fact that violence occurring in taverns was more likely to include more than one person who physically assaulted the respondent (and possibly also other individuals on the side of the respondent). Drunkenness in the principal adversary was imputed by 30% of victims of violence with one adversary ($n = 347$). When more than one adversary victimized the respondent, the proportion was 45% ($n = 47$; $\chi^2 = 4.16$, $df = 1$, $p < .05$).

A tentative descriptive conclusion can be drawn from the findings presented above (and from the similar findings regarding the violent crimes of the community): Drinking is somewhat more common in "brawls" than in other violence. An escalation from a two-person conflict into more inclusive violence may be more likely when alcohol has been used. This circumstance may also be related to the typical public settings in which alcohol is commonly used. The following brief description of violence from the interview survey illustrates the group processes involved in such escalation (in the barest outline):

> "I was at a stag party drinking. Two guys jumped on my friend. I tried to stop them, and one of the fellows bit my finger. My brother kicked the guy in the head so he'd let go of my finger. The two guys left, and I went to the hospital after a few more drinks."

Group proceedings are sometimes helped along by rather familiar conflict-inducing attributions based on ethnicity, nationality, or race, as in these incidents:

> "I was in the States with nine other Canadians. I tried to use Canadian money at a bar, and some Americans told us to go home and said that we were 'stupid Canadians.' We got into a fight, and eventually the cops came and sent us Canadians back to the border."

> "I was coming out of the bathroom in a hotel and a nigger was punching my buddy, so I punched the nigger. Then the nigger got some of his friends and beat me up."

In earlier chapters, I have cited illustrations from the mass media showing the strong ingroup–outgroup character of especially tavern violence: A railway work gang tried to mete out revenge after a few of its

TABLE 6.9. Alcohol Use by the Assailant and Victim Prior to the Most Recent Episode of Physical Violence, as Related to the Number of Assailants and to the Nature and Closeness of the Relationship

	Total alcohol involvement	Drinking by:			
		Assailant	Victim	Both	*Only* assailant
Total sample (*n*'s = 418/451)	54%	51%	30%	26%	22%
Number of assailants					
Only one assailant (*n*'s = 360/382)	52%	49%	28%	25%	23%
More than one assailant (*n*'s = 52/63)	61%	58%	40%	35%	19%
Assailant's relationship to victim					
Spouse (*n*'s = 87/92)	46%	44%	14%	12%	31%
Other family member (*n* = 50)	26%	24%	16%	14%	10%
Good friend (*n*'s = 29/30)	55%	53%	31%	30%	20%
Person known from work, school, or neighborhood (*n*'s = 106/111)	39%	38%	29%	28%	9%
Other casual acquaintance (*n*'s = 25/28)	69%	64%	46%	41%	20%
Extent to which nonfamily assailant known by respondent					
Very well or fairly well (*n*'s = 131/133)	46%	44%	30%	29%	15%
Only a little or hardly at all (*n*'s = 64/71)	50%	47%	32%	29%	16%
Not at all (*n*'s = 102/119)	78%	75%	41%	36%	35%

members were evicted from a local bar (see Chapter 1), and local bar patrons with abundant help from members of the general community attacked a motorcycle gang (as well as its property and one of its pets) in an attempt to dispense justice in another incident (see Chapter 5). From such patterns, interesting theoretical possibilities emerge regarding the determinant interaction between the effects of alcohol and preferred cognitive structurings of situations.

Like the location of any interactional event between two or more individuals, the place where violent episodes occur is associated with *the relationship between the participants*. This association is especially pronounced with regard to interactions between family members, which predominantly occur in the family home. The location of incidents involving other relationships is somewhat less predictable.

I have noted earlier in several contexts that victimization in conjugal violence is much more common in the experience of women than of men. Over half the incidents reported by women were conflicts with their husbands as the assailants, and about two-thirds were instances of family violence, involving a spouse, parent, sibling, or some other relation. The wife was the antagonist in only 7% of the victimizations in violence reported by men, and only 12% were cases of family violence.

Total alcohol involvement was at its highest when physical violence erupted between strangers: In fully three-fourths of such encounters, at least one of the parties involved had consumed some alcohol (Table 6.9). Violence between strangers also involved drinking by both participants more often than in any other relationship, about one-third. Forty-six percent of marital violence occurred after alcohol use by one or both spouses. In a large proportion of these cases, only the assailant (most often the husband) had been drinking.

The serious nature of alcohol use in some marital violence is probably reflected in the finding that divorced or separated respondents had an alcohol involvement of 69% in their most recent subjection to violent acts ($n = 37$), with the antagonist drinking in 65% and the respondent drinking in 35% of these occurrences. In comparison, married respondents had a total alcohol involvement of 49% ($n = 282$), and single respondents 58% ($n = 90$).

In marital violence, the spouse was judged to be "drunk" in 23% of the episodes, while this assessment was made for 56% of total strangers. The amounts of alcohol consumed by the respondents in different relationships can be cited with any degree of reliability only for incidents between strangers. In these the respondents' mean consumption was 9.5 cl of 100% alcohol ($n = 43$), which differs very little from the overall mean of 9.2 cl.

The closeness of a relationship also correlates with reasons and motives for the aggression, acts committed, the private or public resolution of the incident, and so forth. In order to get away to some extent from the qualitative differences between family links and other relationships, I have again omitted family members entirely from some analyses and have only differentiated the relationships by how well known the assailant was to the respondent. This subsample thus consists of violence that occurred between friends, acquaintances, and total strangers, and in a few cases between lovers.

As Table 6.9 shows, there was very little difference in alcohol involvement in violence between nonrelated individuals who knew each other well and violence in which the participants knew each other only little or hardly at all. There were, on the other hand, considerable differences in the presence of alcohol in violence between total strangers and the other two groups. Alcohol was present in over three-fourths of incidents between strangers, but only in about half of the physical aggression between unrelated nonstrangers ($\chi^2 = 21.14$, $df = 1$, $p < .001$). This high level of total alcohol involvement is largely a consequence of the fact that violent strangers were more likely than other assailants to have consumed alcohol. Also, victims had been drinking in a somewhat larger proportion of confrontations with strangers than was the case for other relationships.

The differences in assessed drunkenness of the victimizers were also great: About one-fourth (24%) were judged to be drunk in the episodes where the assailant was known at least to some extent, as compared to 63% for total strangers. There were no significant differences in the mean consumptions of drinking victims in violence between nonrelatives: 9.2 cl for events including nonstrangers ($n = 53$) and 9.6 cl for events involving total strangers ($n = 46$).

It was in marital violence that the assailant was most often the lone drinker, in relative terms (Table 6.9). In part, this can no doubt be accounted for by differences in gender distributions of victimized respondents; I have noted earlier that women were generally much less likely than men to have consumed alcohol in their last victimizations (18% compared to 37% for men; Table 6.6).

SUMMARY OF FINDINGS ON THE PRESENCE OF ALCOHOL IN VIOLENCE

Despite the obvious gaps in the material available on violence that came to the attention of the police and was recorded in occurrence reports, alcohol was noted as having been used prior to 42% of these violent crimes. In comparison, the differently sampled episodes of generally milder forms of violence in the interview study had a total alcohol involvement of 54%. It can thus be said that alcohol was not just present in the most extreme or tragic cases of violence, but was also part of its everyday manifestations. Whatever the biases created by the selection procedures before violent incidents were documented by the authorities, they were correct in showing that alcohol played a major role in violence in this community; this is probably also true of many other similar communities and wider geographical areas.

In the interview material, the low rate of drinking by the victim alone, compared to the much higher level of alcohol use only by the assailant, indicated that alcohol had a central effect in instigating physical violence. Another general observation is that the police record data seemed generally to reflect patterns of problem drinking in both offenders and victims to a much greater extent than was the case for violence accessed through interviews with the general population.

Drinking was a predominantly male activity in this community, and so was drinking prior to violence (by both victims and assailants). In the interview population, alcohol involvement was highest among assailants and victims in their 20s, whereas the violent crimes showed higher involvement in older age groups; perhaps this is another indication of the greater presence of problem drinkers in this set of data. An increasing proportion of alcohol in violence was evident with increasing age among teenage victims and (to a somewhat lesser extent) among teenage offenders in violent crime.

Drinking was more common in violence with more than two participants. This was evident from both the police data on violent crimes and the interview information on violence. Group violence was more saturated with alcohol than violence in clearly discernible dyads.

In both sources of data, marital violence and domestic violence generally showed the well-documented pattern of a drinking assailant (with few exceptions, the husband) and a sober victim. In fact, the rates were almost identical between the two sources. In the interview data, violence between strangers was more strongly related to drinking than violence in any other type of relationship. This was not the case in violent crimes, where marital violence had the highest rate of drinking of all known relationships.

Amounts of alcohol consumed by the victims (available only in the interview data) were generally greater when they were subjected to violence than in the common drinking situations in the community. However, these former volumes were considerably smaller than the same persons' maximum amount consumed in the past 30 days (for infrequent drinkers, the last 12 months). Very few of the peak drinking events had led to angry arousal in a drinker, and hardly any to the use of physical force on the part of the drinker (these findings are not discussed in this book). It is evident that other contingencies must be present for drinking to result in the instigation of open conflict and violence. The interactions between alcohol effects and these contingencies in the determination of open aggression should be a central focus in the study of the connections between drinking and violence.

In this chapter, we have seen some instances of expanded possibilities for analysis when a survey method is used for studying alcohol's relationship with violence. For the next two chapters, the official documents fall short, and the analyses therefore rely entirely on data collected through interviews. Chapter 7 examines the types of violent acts perpetrated by the assailants, and Chapter 8 looks at the outcomes of these acts in the form of injuries and medical attention to the injuries.

7

Violent Acts: Determinants of Choice

In earlier chapters, the characteristics of actors and settings in violent episodes have been described, as has the presence of alcohol in relation to these characteristics. This chapter examines the types of violent acts used by the assailants in aggression against the victims. The linkages between the choice of acts on the one hand, and the characteristics of the participants, the settings, and (above all) the connections to drinking on the other, are studied. No reliable descriptions of what violent acts were used were available in the occurrence reports of police, and thus only data from the interview study have been used in the analyses presented here.[1]

In examining the influence of alcohol use on the choice of acts, and, in the next chapter, on injuries sustained by the victim, I briefly touch upon theoretical issues that have been studied almost exclusively through

1. It is difficult to imagine any reliable methodology that does not in some way directly use the recollections of participants in physical violence for this purpose, be they victims, assailants, or witnesses. Variations are possible in the selection of sampling frames and respondents (e.g., interviews could be conducted with or questionnaires filled out by participants in officially detected violence, by victims showing up at health care centers or emergency rooms, etc.). The possibilities of experimental simulations seem very limited. These are currently focused on measures of the frequency and intensity of and perseverance in one and the same very specific type of act—usually pushing a button graded as to its intensity of electric shock. This is a semiotically and transactionally very circumscribed aggressive act, with no close precedents in real life, and it would seem that the subjects must actively define and project any such social dimensions into their behavior in the experimental setting. They are often helped along by "cover stories" told or "cover tasks" presented to them by the experimenter. However, parallel and complementary analyses based on real-life sources are needed.

experimental methodology. Such experiments typically compare subjects who have been drinking and subjects who have not in the extent of aggressive reactions to stimuli that are intended to be threatening, frustrating, provoking, or generally stressful to the subjects. Although the present study's retrospectively sampled episodes of violence are fraught with the problems of a post hoc methodology, it is important to try to test hypotheses conceived in experimental thinking with real-life material. In this way, it may be possible to bridge the unnecessarily large gap between experimental research and social research efforts attempting to study the same empirical phenomena.

I also briefly touch upon the two main explanatory frames of human conduct that have been discussed in the first chapter: the frame of the consciously guided and that of the naturally caused. We have seen earlier how the two frames compete especially acutely when intoxicated behavior is perceived and explained. The natural frame seems to have had the upper hand, probably due in part to alcohol's status as a pharmacologically active substance, whereas researchers stressing thematic guidedness have severely attacked this conceptualization.

GENERAL HYPOTHESES REGARDING ALCOHOL'S ROLE IN HUMAN AGGRESSION

First, however, I give a brief presentation of three of the most common clusters of hypotheses regarding the determinant role of alcohol in human aggression. These clusters underlie theoretical discussions in the area of alcohol and aggressive behavior. Only two of these are directly addressed here through an analysis of empirical data, but the third group of hypotheses is potentially so central that it deserves our attention despite the lack of testing material.

Severity and Persistence Hypotheses

First, the "severity" hypothesis argues that with alcohol use, aggressive acts will become more severe or extreme. This type of hypothesis has been tested in many experimental studies, where severity has been measured by the intensity of electric shock settings (allegedly) administered to other subjects (e.g., Bennett, Buss, & Carpenter, 1969; Gustafson, 1986a; Lang, Goeckner, Adesso, & Marlatt, 1975; Pihl, Smith, & Farrell, 1984; Taylor, Schmutte, & Leonard, 1977). Related to this idea is the "persistence" hypothesis, or the assumption that acts of aggression will be more persistent after the use of alcohol. The persistence of aggression has been measured by, for example, the duration of shock (although often this has not been conceptually distinguished from a purportedly general measure of aggression in experimental paradigms).

There are some indications from the experimental literature that severity and persistence are functionally independent, in that alcohol shows different determinant patterns on shock intensity than on shock duration in some experiments. This distinction is not of great concern in regard to the present study, since types of acts used by the assailants and injuries caused to the victim are conceived of as indicators of a more global concept of severity of violence. In a more analytical vein, such a general concept has been established through pooling numbers of shocks given and the measures of intensity and duration of shocks in order to arrive at a single general measure of aggression (Gustafson, 1986b).

A real-life corollary of both the severity and persistence hypotheses is that more violent acts will be committed and that rates and extent of injuries will be more serious when the assailants have been drinking than would be the case under similar conditions when the assailants are sober. Some data pertaining to violent crime have been used to test this hypothesis, and they have generally supported it (Roslund & Larson, 1979; Tardif, 1967; Wolfgang, 1958). The number of *different types* of physically violent acts perpetrated could be used as an indicator of persistence in the present study, but this measure has been looked at only sporadically in the analyses. Systematic tests have been carried out using types of violent acts and probability of physical injury as indicators of the severity of violence.

Indiscrimination Hypotheses

The "indiscrimination" hypotheses state that acts of aggression after drinking will not be as well attuned as acts of sober aggression to the requirements of the situation and the social norms applying to it, such as the restraints (or "inhibitions") related to the location, the types of acts performed, the characteristics of the target of aggression, and so forth. Thus, strictures against serious violence in the presence of witnesses, against women and children, and so on would not be as evident after alcohol use, and acts performed would be as serious as in other social contexts, regardless of the presence of normally attenuating factors. Experimental paradigms have used some victim characteristics and victim behaviors as discriminating cues. Thus, Zeichner and Pihl (1980) measured the effect of expressed intent by an (alleged) adversary on the aggression of drinking and nondrinking subjects; Schmutte and Taylor (1980) varied pain feedback from a decoy victim; and Yankofsky, Wilson, Adler, Hay, and Vrana (1986) used neutral versus negative feedback from a confederate for discriminatory purposes. The findings generally indicate more indiscriminateness and insensitivity to empirical contingencies after alcohol use in the evaluation of feedback and in the aggression committed.

Possible extensions within this theoretical indiscrimination theme could include hypotheses regarding displacement of aggression, measuring the variability in the target of aggression in addition to the variability of the nature of the aggression; if no other alcohol-specific processes intervene (a much more voluminous "if" than it might seem to be), one might, for example, expect that another person or object would more readily become the target of aggression after alcohol use if the original target for some reason is or becomes unavailable. No doubt indiscrimination hypotheses, as well as the more specific alcohol-linked displacement hypotheses, can be tested experimentally more directly and systematically than has hitherto been the case.

Elicitation Hypotheses

The third group of hypotheses that can be derived from the literature addresses alcohol-related aggressive processes that sequentially precede the processes covered by the other two groups. These are the "elicitation" hypotheses. A general elicitation hypothesis would state that given any social situation (or any specified range of such situations, such as ones that contain provoking, threatening, or frustrating cues), a person or persons using alcohol are more likely to engage in conflict, aggression, and violence than are sober actors in an equivalent situation. In other words, adding alcohol use to any situation (or a specified range of situations) will lead to a greater risk of eliciting aggressive reactions. (Alternatively, this type of hypothesis could be referred to as an "incitement" or "instigation" hypothesis.)

We can also speak of an "indiscrimination-in-elicitation" hypothesis (as opposed to, e.g. an "indiscrimination-in-response" hypothesis), in that (objective and/or phenomenologically conceived) cues in a situation that under sober circumstances would not lead to a higher risk of aggression and violence will do so under the influence of alcohol. Experimental findings indicate at least a lower threshold (very figuratively speaking) for the effects of instigating cues after the use of alcohol, be they frustrative, threatening, or provocative (e.g., Gustafson, 1986a; Taylor, Gammon, & Capasso, 1976; Zeichner & Pihl, 1979). However, these effects are usually measured in terms of severity and persistence, since typically no nonaggressive response alternatives are provided to the subject.

In anecdotal real-life material pertaining to drunken aggression, the changes in elicitation processes can be detected in the form of the *trifling* nature of the circumstances that seem to bring about drunken wrath and aggression. This indicates a difference in the sensitization to environmental cues or stimulus generalization of cues, categorizations, and responses after drinking. What seems to be most basically missing from the experimental agenda is the *ad libitum* condition, or free choice of behavior cues: Does intoxication increase the risk that aggression-eliciting cues (among other cues in the situation) will be perceived, attended to, and/or recognized as such? (On the face of it, this would seem to go against the lack of discrimination that has been found for other types of behavior cues; on the other hand, it seems in part supported by findings implying greater discrimination between threatening and nonthreatening cues, as well as between frustrating and non frustrating cues, etc.) This embryonic cluster of hypotheses linked to elicitation is important because hardly any of elicitation's many possible roles in the explanation of drunken aggression have been studied in an analytical manner, although it seems to be implicit in much of the discussion on how alcohol may lead to aggressive behavior. It seems that a study of real-life episodes would very nicely complement experimental studies of this question. The material presented in this book does not enable us to evaluate any limits of the validity of a general elicitation or instigation hypothesis. (Plans are under way for such research, however).

There are other clusters of empirical openings in the ideal "instigation–arousal–aggression–physical violence" sequence in which alcohol may exert its effects on characteristics of aggression and violence. One such is the emergent idea that alcohol has its main influence in the choice-of-response stage (Steele & Southwick, 1985). It is important to note that these different types of hypotheses do not necessarily contradict one another; most of them actually do not, since they apply to different stages of the aggression sequence and to different empirical contingencies. They may in fact all be true, and the hypothesized processes may all be active in producing characteristics of intoxicated aggression, given suitable constellations of empirical factors.

This chapter presents some partial tests of the severity and the indiscrimination hypotheses, based on the episode sample from the interview study. However, I am also concerned in part here with the descriptive groundwork of the relationship between alcohol use and aggression. It bears repeating that the present research and analyses should ideally be of relevance for closing the unnecessarily great gap between social and psychological research methodology and the theoretical work inspired by these methodologies.

ACTS, ADVERSARIES, AND SETTINGS

Events and sequences of events that incorporate physical violence of one type or another can differ greatly with regard to the characteristics of actors involved, the settings in which the violence occurs, the imputed reasons for the conflict, the types of violence perpetrated, the situational resolutions or outcomes, the extent of injuries, the damage to relationships, legal consequences, and so forth. The variability of reasons, settings, actors, and outcomes in such a seemingly unitary phenomenon as physical aggression is evident from the following selection of incidents briefly related by the residents of Thunder Bay when describing their most recent victimizations:

"The kids were laughing and my husband had a temper. The more he told them to stop, the more they laughed, so he hit me because I couldn't get them to stop. Nothing was said after that. I never answered back."

"I was living with my brother. I was 16 and he was 17. He was always partying and hanging out with a rough crowd. I got up Christmas morning and had to clean up the mess, and I objected. He pushed me and I fell into the tub."

"I was gathered with a group and we were talking, and this police guard came and ordered us to spread out and we didn't move fast enough, so I got a shaking up."

"A friend of mine and I had both been in the army. It seemed that I had got the better of him in a fight in the past, and now his brother wanted to prove that he was better than his brother. There was a fight, and I lost a couple of teeth, but I came out best in the end. I have never seen him since."

"A bunch of us, boys and girls, were in the park one night, and some other boys came along and didn't like us being with those girls, and they started fighting us. Finally, after some bleeding, the fighting stopped."

"I let my friend get ahead of me in the line. The person behind me didn't like it, and we exchanged a few words. And then the man hit me. I called the man outside, and we had a pretty rough fight. The police came and broke it up."

"It started because some fellows tried to rape me. I won the fight. I kicked and fought, and finally they left me alone."

"I was a policeman at the time. We received a call that a man was wrecking a house. We tried to arrest him—it took three policemen. In the scuffle I was hit with a chair. The man was arrested."

"I was dancing with another fellow's girl, and he told me to get away, but she refused to let me. He got one of his friends to help him, and they grabbed me, and one of them stabbed me with a small knife."

"I was walking with my friend, and two guys came up to me and hit me with something sharp. They tried to steal my wallet and punched me and broke my nose. Some other people came by, and the guys took off."

"I came in from the club late, and my wife had kept dinner waiting for 2 hours. She hit me with a frying pan. I got kind of dizzy, but my wife was worse off. She had to go to the hospital to get 87 stitches in her hand, because it went through a stained-glass window when she struck at me."

"I was down in the bar and went to my hotel room. I left the door open when I was in the bathroom. When I returned there was a man behind the door. He hit me with a crowbar. I passed out, and he left."

Ideally, the number of individual acts of violence committed by the assailant, the force of the acts, and other details about the nature of the violence, as well as the injuries sustained, should be considered in determining the seriousness of violence and testing composite severity and indiscrimination hypotheses. In addition to the number of punches, for example, we should know where on the body the respondent was hit; what type of weapon or object was used; whether the respondent was grabbed around the throat or only on the arm; whether the grabbing only involved holding or also twisting the arm; what type of pushing act was involved (e.g., out of a room, against a wall, down on the floor, or down a flight of stairs); whether the violence continued despite obvious injury to the victim or to both adversaries; and so on. This type of information would enable us to make more refined operationalizations of the apparent seriousness and intent to hurt. It would also help in determining assailants' discrimination or lack of discrimination regarding the type of violence and force that was allowed or required in a certain type of situation and with a specific type of victim. Simple information on the duration of the altercation or beating, as well as patterns of escalation, de-escalation, and recurring flareups, would likewise aid us in theorizing about violence and the role of alcohol in it. Were we able to follow the whole process of interaction, we might detect important perspectives on the instrumental, communicational, and generally transactional functions of violent acts and the ways in which alcohol influences these. In the present study, with the relatively small sample sizes involved, the lack of previous investigations of many central variables that could guide assessments of their relevance, and limitations imposed by competing objectives, such detail had to be left for future endeavors.[2]

Common Types and Combinations of Types of Violence

Community residents were subjected to only one type of violent act in 63% of their most recent violent encounters (see questions 3 and 6 of Appendix B, or Table 7.1 below, for the categories of acts presented by means of a flash card to respondents). Sixty percent of the violence directed against men consisted of one type of act only, compared to 66% for women—a difference that was not statistically significant. A slightly greater proportion of women than men were subjected to a high number of different types of violence on the same occasion; 5.1% of women and 3.7% of men were victims of at least five of the listed types of acts in the same episode. The corresponding shares of at least six different types of acts were 2.2% and 1.0%. This pattern of greater concentration of aggression among relatively few female victims is reminiscent of that found earlier for the numbers of threats and violence episodes experienced during a 12-month period. Here, the difference was well within the bounds of sampling fluctuations, however.

Punching (hitting with clenched fist) and slapping were the most common single types of victimizations. Eighteen percent of the most recent victimizations were such that only punching was involved on the part of the assailant; in 16% the victim was only slapped; and in another 14% only grabbing, pushing, or shoving was used against the victim. The percentages for the other types of acts when used singly were considerably lower, ranging between 3% and 5%. The weapons or objects used for hitting varied widely (knives, pieces of wood, beer bottles, broken beer glasses, brass knuckles, a crowbar, a car, etc.). The "other violent acts" category similarly included a very varied range of violent behavior (being shot at, "sexually attacked," choked, tripped, bitten, burned with a cigarette, scratched, pulled by the hair, etc.).

The proportions of the different acts that were combined with at least one other type of violent act in the same violence episode were as follows:

2. An in-depth study of violent crime events through interviews with offenders and/or victims could form one starting point. (As stated earlier, records of violent crime kept by police and other authorities are too uneven in coverage, unreliable in quality, and lacking in detail for such purposes). Another simple device (as part of broad strategy) would be to let respondents rate the seriousness of the episodes where physical violence was used by asking, for instance, whether they felt in danger of their lives, in danger of getting hurt, and the like.

Hitting with weapon or object: 72% ($n = 69$)
Punching/hitting with fist: 60% ($n = 194$)
Kicking: 76% ($n = 91$)
Throwing of object: 71% ($n = 52$)
Slapping: 57% ($n = 162$)
Grabbing, pushing, or shoving: 61% ($n = 158$)
Other violent acts: 55% ($n = 31$)

These proportions probably reflect, among other things, the extent to which certain types of violence are part of an escalatory pattern. Regarding punching/hitting with fist, there was a gender-specific pattern that may reflect differences in the normative expectations guiding this violent behavior. Among female victims, the proportion of combinations that included punching was 79% ($n = 42$), whereas it was 55% ($n = 152$) among men. The difference was significant on the .02 level ($\chi^2 = 6.52$, $df = 1$). This indicates that punching a woman with the fist may more often be part of an escalatory pattern and not an attempt at instant subjugation or injury. This would imply in turn that cross-gender violence may have more of the characteristics of negotiated interactions, where normatively motivated lines are drawn and sometimes crossed, where the meanings of violent acts are acutely questioned and defined, and where lasting implications for the relationship are continually at the fore.

A converse pattern emerged for grabbing, pushing, or shoving, which was more often combined with other violent acts among male (71%; $n = 72$) than among female (52%; $n = 88$) victims ($\chi^2 = 4.96$, $df = 1$, $p < .05$). This may be connected to the predominantly intimate nature of grabbing, pushing, and shoving, and the fact that they occur in the context of different motives for conflict and different relationships in all-male and cross-gender violence. In conflicts between males, this relatively mild form of violence may be part of an escalatory (or de-escalatory) pattern, in which concerns over proprieties regarding "too intimate" violent acts give way to more instrumental concerns about coming out on top (or putting an end to more dangerous acts). In violent conflict between a man and a woman, the instrumental, communicational, or transactional aims may be met more often through these types of acts without recourse to other violence. There were no significant differences between victimized men and women in the prevalence of combinations that included the other types of violent acts.

Gender-Related Patterns

The types of violent acts (as well as the resolutions and outcomes of the violence) differed greatly between individual episodes. Some very distinct patterns could be discerned for different groups of victims, though. Acts

TABLE 7.1. Violent Acts Committed Against the Victim in the Most Recent Episode of Physical Violence, as Related to Characteristics of the Victim, Assailant, and Setting

	Hitting with weapon/object	Punching	Kicking	Throwing an object	Slapping	Grabbing, pushing, or shoving	Other violent acts
Total ($n = 450$)	15%	43%	20%	12%	36%	36%	7%
Gender of victim							
Male ($n = 267$)	18%	57%	25%	8%	26%	27%	7%
Female ($n = 183$)	11%	23%	14%	18%	50%	48%	7%
Gender of assailant							
Male ($n = 372$)	16%	48%	22%	11%	31%	36%	7%
Female ($n = 73$)	12%	23%	10%	14%	61%	33%	9%
Age of victim							
Under 30 ($n = 279$)	17%	43%	20%	11%	36%	32%	7%
30 and over ($n = 161$)	12%	43%	21%	12%	34%	42%	6%
Age of assailant							
Under 30 ($n = 278$)	15%	46%	21%	10%	33%	32%	7%
30 and over ($n = 164$)	15%	40%	17%	13%	41%	41%	7%

Location of violence							
Own home ($n = 155$)	11%	23%	11%	17%	56%	39%	4%
Other private home ($n = 47$)	7%	42%	20%	2%	47%	36%	9%
Work or school ($n = 67$)	17%	53%	32%	12%	29%	37%	6%
Public drinking place ($n = 75$)	22%	62%	30%	6%	22%	29%	5%
Street or park ($n = 60$)	19%	47%	26%	11%	10%	37%	13%
Other location ($n = 42$)	19%	60%	15%	12%	22%	33%	12%
Relationship of assailant to victim							
Spouse ($n = 90$)	10%	30%	11%	20%	61%	42%	6%
Other family member ($n = 50$)	10%	14%	12%	6%	52%	28%	4%
Friend/acquaintance ($n = 166$)	16%	46%	20%	11%	32%	35%	5%
Stranger ($n = 124$)	18%	60%	28%	7%	18%	37%	11%
Spouse *or* other family member[a] ($n = 140$)	10%	24%	11%	15%	58%	37%	5%
Extent to which assailant known[b]							
Very well or fairly well ($n = 115$)	14%	42%	20%	12%	44%	29%	5%
A little or hardly at all ($n = 70$)	18%	59%	24%	4%	20%	37%	6%
Not at all ($n = 120$)	18%	58%	28%	8%	19%	36%	11%
Number of assailants							
One ($n = 381$)	15%	40%	17%	12%	38%	36%	7%
More than one ($n = 64$)	16%	63%	38%	10%	23%	35%	10%

[a]Note that this category is the sum of the first two relationship categories.
[b]The "spouse or other family member" category is not included.

directed against women typically differed from acts to which men were subjected (Table 7.1). Punching ($\chi^2 = 51.13$, $df = 1$, $p < .001$), kicking ($\chi^2 = 7.82$, $df = 1$, $p < .01$), and hitting with a weapon or object ($\chi^2 = 4.27$, $df = 1$, $p < .05$) were acts predominantly experienced by male victims when violence occurred, whereas slapping ($\chi^2 = 26.96$, $df = 1$, $p < .001$), grabbing, pushing, or shoving ($\chi^2 = 21.09$, $df = 1$, $p < .001$), and the throwing of objects ($\chi^2 = 10.54$, $df = 1, p < .01$) were much more typical experiences of women. Women probably experienced more violence of a sexual nature than did men; this would explain the higher proportion of acts in the grabbing, pushing, or shoving category.

Male and female subjections to combinations of different types of acts are shown in Table 7.2 for the 11 most common combinations. As stated earlier, the most common single act was punching, followed by slapping and the disjunctive category of grabbing, pushing, or shoving. Among the events in which the respondents were subjected to two types of acts, the most common combination was punching combined with slapping (5% of all incidents). Punching together with kicking or with grabbing, pushing, or shoving had a prevalence of 3%, as did the latter category combined with slapping. The above-mentioned four types of acts also appeared together in the most common three- and four-type combinations.

The most common victimization experience in violence among men was being punched by the adversary with no other types of acts involved; no doubt, in a great proportion of cases, this was a fistfight with another man. This single category made up over one-fourth of the last violent occurrences among men, but only 1 in 20 among women ($\chi^2 = 33.44$, $df = 1, p < .001$). Incidents that consisted only of slapping made up 23% of victimizations among women, compared to 11% among men ($\chi^2 = 11.91$, $df = 1$, $p < .001$). Grabbing, pushing, or shoving alone occurred in another 23% of female experiences of violence; in only 8% of episodes was this true for men ($\chi^2 = 20.33$, $df = 1, p < .001$). These two generally milder forms of violence thus made up 46% of female experiences and 19% of male experiences. Conversely, men had a much higher proportion of events in which at least one relatively severe type of act was included, as might be expected from the findings regarding separate acts (see Table 7.1). (The next chapter looks directly at the seriousness of acts by examining the extent to which community residents reported being injured in these violent encounters and the extent to which they sought medical care.)

I have already noted that female victims were much less likely to have been punched with a clenched fist than were male victims. Table 7.1 also shows that women as perpetrators of violence were much less likely to punch ($\chi^2 = 15.36$, $df = 1$, $p < .001$) and kick ($\chi^2 = 6.05$, $df = 1$,

$p < .05$) their opponents, and much more likely to slap them ($\chi^2 = 25.16$, $df = 1$, $p < .001$).

A central finding is that women tended to be subjected to types of violence that they were themselves likely to use against others (and that they also were more likely to have witnessed—see Chapter 4). This cannot be explained by women's being disproportionately often victimized by other women; as we shall see later, this pattern of violence was also found when men victimized women. Even physical violence seems to be governed by rules or norms, and interactional restrictions on violence falling under a general "tit-for-tat" or reciprocity rule appear to be at play here. This finding is an indication of the important fact that aggression and violence do not typically just spring from the perpetrator and are not exclusively or even predominantly determined by his/her characteristics and acute mental state, such as a rageful or "disinhibited" state. In the majority of cases, violence is rule-governed interaction—a species of "guided doing." There are very serious exceptions to guidance by such rules and limits, of course, and these cases disproportionately end up being documented by the police, the courts, and the mass media.

Age-Related Tendencies

Violence experienced before the age of 30 and after that age differed remarkably little (Table 7.1)—much less so than violence experienced by the two genders. The only notable difference (10 percentage points) was for grabbing, pushing, or shoving, which was experienced relatively more often in violence after age 30 ($\chi^2 = 5.06$, $df = 1$, $p < .05$). Dividing the sample into four age categories (under 20, 20–29, 30–39, and 40 and over) did not reveal any significant patterns, either, except that slapping tended to be less common in the oldest age group.

Assailants aged 30 and over resorted more often to both slapping and grabbing, pushing, or shoving (Table 7.1). Both differences only reached the .10 level of significance, however. It may be concluded very cautiously that more serious acts decrease marginally with age, while less serious ones show a marginal increase. Further breakdowns indicated that these slight tendencies were mainly due to age-related patterns among female victims (results not shown).

Location-Related Patterns

There were great differences in the types of violent acts used in different types of locations (Table 7.1). In the home setting, punching and kicking were far less common than average, whereas slapping in particular was more prevalent. Taverns and bars were the locations highest in compara-

TABLE 7.2 Combinations of Violent Acts Committed Against the Victim in the Most Recent Episode of Physical Violence, by Gender of Victim

Combination	Male victim (n = 265)	Female victim (n = 182)	Total (n = 447)
Only punching	26%	5%	18%
Only slapping	11%	23%	16%
Only grabbing, pushing, or shoving	8%	23%	14%
Only kicking	5%	4%	5%
Both punching *and* slapping	5%	4%	5%
Only hitting with weapon/object	6%	2%	4%
Only throwing of object	2%	5%	3%
Both punching *and* grabbing, pushing, or shoving	6%	0%	3%
Only other violent acts	3%	3%	3%
Both slapping *and* grabbing, pushing, or shoving	1%	6%	3%
Both punching *and* kicking	5%	0%	3%
Other combinations	23%	25%	24%

Note. Percentages in some columns may not total 100% because of rounding.

tively serious acts of violence: Public drinking places had the highest proportions of hitting with a weapon or object and of hitting with fists, as well as the second highest rate of kicking. The two potentially least harmful types of acts—slapping and grabbing, pushing, or shoving—had relatively low frequencies in drinking establishments.

Other Patterns

As a rule, the less close the relationship between the adversaries in violence, the more common hitting and kicking became (Table 7.1). Still, it is noteworthy that about one-third of marital violence included hitting the victim with a fist. Tentative comparisons between male and female victims as to the prevalence of acts in physically violent incidents are possible for two central relationships: spouses and total strangers (Table 7.3).

Acts directed at the husband and the wife in marital violence differed remarkably little except for the category of grabbing, pushing, or shoving. This similarity again shows that violent interactions may generally be governed by reciprocity norms in such relationships. There are physical limitations to the application of such a rule with regard to grabbing (or holding) and shoving (including wrestling matches, etc.), and a woman's generally smaller size and lesser strength may stop her from trying these acts. These acts are also typical of sexually motivated violence, and as such will be directed more against women than men.

TABLE 7.3. Violent Acts Committed against Victims by Spouses and Strangers in the Most Recent Episode of Physical Violence, by Gender of Victim

	Spouse as assailant		Stranger as assailant	
Type of violence	Male victim ($n = 16$)	Female victim ($n = 74$)	Male victim ($n = 101$)	Female victim ($n = 23$)
Hitting with weapon or object	13%	10%	22%	0%
Punching/hitting with fist	31%	30%	67%	26%
Kicking	6%	12%	31%	17%
Throwing an object	13%	22%	6%	9%
Slapping	69%	60%	17%	22%
Grabbing, pushing or shoving	6%	50%	30%	70%
Other violent acts	6%	5%	9%	17%

When the assailant was a total stranger, there were more pronounced differences between acts endured by men and women. Needless to say, the small number of cases in two of the columns of Table 7.3 make the findings very tentative and in need of verification in larger samples. There was a slight tendency for more severe violent acts to be used when the adversaries did not know each other well, and a definite tendency for especially slapping to be used less (Table 7.1). To some extent, again, this is no doubt due to the greater proportion of women victimized in close relationships. Multivariate procedures have been used to address this question (see "Determinant Patterns in Acts of Violence," below).

Acts of physical violence tended to be more forceful and potentially more dangerous to the victim when there was more than one assailant (Table 7.1). This was markedly true for kicking ($\chi^2 = 14.66$, $df = 1$, $p < .001$) and punching ($\chi^2 = 11.05$, $df = 1, p < .001$). Slapping was less common with multiple assailants ($\chi^2 = 6.03$, $df = 1, p < .02$). The mean number of different types of violent acts was also greater when two or more persons victimized the respondent (1.92 compared to 1.64).

THE RULE-GOVERNED GUIDEDNESS OF HUMAN VIOLENCE: AN INTERMEDIARY DISCUSSION

As noted more than once above, violent acts directed against women generally differed from the acts to which men were subjected. In fact, a central conclusion from the analyses described to this point can be summarized as follows: Acts of violence are determined more by the gender of the target than by the gender of the perpetrator. The results have also shown that the location of a violent incident is strongly linked to the aggressive acts perpetrated. Taken together, these conclusions suggest that *in the determination of physical violence, the constellation of victim and setting is more important than are the characteristics of the perpetrator alone.* There are no doubt extreme cases and perpetrators of violence for which and whom this pattern of determination does not hold true, but within this general population of subjects it can be inferred from the empirical facts. What most essentially distinguishes "pathological" (or "deviant") incidents of violence from everyday violence may in fact be the much greater obliviousness toward or disregard for characteristics of setting and adversary—a seemingly wanton indiscrimination of rules and normatively relevant factors. Wife battering and physical child abuse are tragic examples of violence in which commonly accepted interactional rules and transactional meanings of aggressive acts are totally disregarded, and probably replaced by more idiosyncratic determination. A later section of this chapter examines the effects alcohol use may have as a modifier of this commonly multifactorial, symbolic, interactional, and communicational determination.

The fact that gender of the victim determines the violent acts carried out to a greater extent than does the gender of the assailant thus indicates that the interactional setup and the subjective meanings attached to this constellation are very important. This is not just a question of normative determination; other semiotic processes evolve in part *within* the frames provided by cultural or subcultural norms. For instance, by carrying out a violent act a person defines himself to the victim, to any witnesses, and to himself in the constantly ongoing definitions and redefinitions of self, others, and reality (Powers, 1986). (Generally, such definitions form a great part of human existence, since this existence is largely based on symbolic structures establishing meaning and irrelevance; (see Berger & Luckmann, 1966.) In most cases the perpetrator is acutely aware of this definitional dimension of his aggressive behavior, although it is more often than not phrased in such conventional individualistic and moral terms as "responsibility," "concern," and "pity," especially in after-the-fact accounts of the episode. Being aware, the perpetrator also modifies his behavior accordingly. In some circumstances, this type of social defining and/or socially expressive process will lead to a tendency toward less serious forms of violence and attenuation of consequences; in other cases it will result in an exacerbation. The present task, in part, turns into finding out how alcohol use affects this feedback process in natural situations. This is part of the analytical agenda aimed at studying the possible "indiscrimination" of violence after alcohol use, although the determinant processes are more emphatically symbolic, definitional, and cultural than the paradigm of stimulus–response or cue-related determination, within which the concept of discrimination–indiscrimination has been explicated, would lead us to believe.

Humans select certain forms of behavior, types of aggression, and acts of violence partly for their symbolic impact on adversaries and, in many cases, on bystanders. The impact will be different in different settings and with different adversaries. (This process and its outcomes is of course greatly determined by the feedback received in the situation from the adversaries and the bystanders.) Hurting or injuring the opponent will most often be secondary to "making a point" or to achieving other, more transparently instrumental objectives, such as coercion. But, quite as importantly, one can also (try to) make a very definite point through hurting or injuring an antagonist. We get closer to unraveling the determinant patterns in violence by studying the meaningful points to be made than by, for example, merely classifying acts according to their severity and concentrating on the amount of hurt or injury delivered. Through a specific act, even (or especially) one that is physically violent in nature, a human being may say any of the following: "I don't want this to go any further," "I am willing to stand my ground," "I have had enough of this," or, in the right context and phase of violent interaction, even "Mom and Dad are not really angry at each other." *A violent act is usually a "guided doing" of the type that characterizes human behavior in general.* The natural-paradigms that have dominated explanations of behavior under the influence of alcohol neglect these processes, and implicitly assume that they do not apply after (sufficient) alcohol use. Again, a later section of this chapter uses the present empirical data to examine whether these rules persist or whether indiscrimination of target and setting and increased severity are characteristic of alcohol-related violence in this general population.

The semiotic dimensions of violence may be illustrated with the act of throwing an object. (I have noted above that 8% of men and 18% of women had last been victimized through the use of this act [Table 7.1], and that the difference was significant on the .01 level.) The starting point is this: Violence aimed at women was generally proscribed in this community. This was evident from responses to the following statement presented to the interviewees: "Under no circumstances does a man have the right to beat his wife" (item o, question 2, Appendix B). Eighty-four percent of men and 89% of women in the community agreed "mostly" or "completely" with this statement. The existence of such a strong norm may be linked to the comparatively great proportion of throwing of objects at women, and may thus have theoretical implications for the transactional dimensions of violence. The throwing of an object at another person is probably as much a gesture of a communicational nature as it is an act of violence with the intent to hurt the target. First, a man who is using a projectile is not actually "laying hands" on a woman, thereby absolving himself of some of the negative definitions of self that may be generated and applied by himself, the target, and other persons possibly observing the episode. Second, it is in part left up to chance whether the object thrown actually hits the target. There may even be a case—useful for rationalizations and the denial of serious intent, and serviceable as a hedge against accusations of deliberate breach of rules—for claiming that the target is partly at fault for not moving away or ducking from the symbolically intended missile.

In this context, it is of some interest to note that a majority of community residents (close to two-thirds) thought that what other people in general, and family and friends in particular, would think or say was an important reason for most people to avoid physically hurting another person even when aroused to grave anger (Table 7.4). The question was phrased as follows: "What do you think stops most people from physically hurting another person even when they are really angry?" (see question 109 in Appendix B). It is a fairly safe guess that had the question asked specifically about engaging in violence against a woman, this proportion would have been still higher. Fear of getting hurt and respect or fear of the law, as well as moral qualms about violence, were seen as important reasons for nonviolence by a greater proportion of city residents, but this is not of central concern in the present context. Women seemed to interpret the reluctance to engage in violence more in terms of social desirability and moral qualms, whereas there was no difference between genders in assigning fear of injury or fear of legal authorities an important role. The same types of considerations probably explain some aspects of behavior when violence is actually taking place.

TABLE 7.4. Proportions of Men and Women Who Felt That Selected Reasons Were Important in Stopping People from Physically Hurting Someone Else Even When Really Angry

Reason	Men ($n = 512$)	Women ($n = 465$)	Total ($n = 977$)
Because they are concerned about what people who see them will think	57%	66%	61%
Because they are concerned about what their friends will say	58%	69%	63%
Because they are concerned about what their family will say	62%	72%	67%
Because they are afraid of getting hurt themselves	72%	71%	71%
Because they do not want to get into trouble with the law	87%	88%	88%
Because they feel violence is wrong	73%	80%	77%

Some incidents of physical violence consist of a single act of violence without any preceding interaction and escalation. Such episodes also often lack a resolution that would explain the act or provide cognitive context and closure to the incident in other ways. They leave the victim perplexed even after several years have passed, as in this example: "I was standing in a crowded train, and this person ground a lighted cigarette into my hand. I just stood there stunned, and the person left."

At the other extreme are occurrences that last over an extended period of time, with distinct patterns of escalation and de-escalation and clear reciprocity rules. (Some long-lasting relationships that include violent behavior should be viewed as such sequences, with considerable carryover from one aggressive episode to the next. Family feuds display this type of structuring of behavior over generations and with interchangeable actors.) Sometimes sheer luck or chance determines the final outcome without anything that can be called a resolution to the satisfaction of either party—for example, the police arrive, or one party is forced for other reasons to leave town. One aspect of "deviance disavowal" in connection with drunken behavior is that a case is made for not applying reciprocity rules, and for preventing transepisodic carryover of violence ("I was drunk and out of my mind—no hard feelings?"). MacAndrew and Edgerton (1969) cite several instances of such rule invalidations justified by drinking in different cultures.

Some acts in an aggression episode will be part of an escalatory pattern; others are part of a de-escalatory sequel. Sometimes these will form a fluctuating pattern of escalation and de-escalation in one and the same sequence. Such patterns and variations of these are rather nicely illustrated in many a National Hockey League (NHL) game, where fist fights, wrestling matches, and free-for-alls may alternate over periods of 10 minutes or more, with relatively calm moments interspersed with flareups. Hockey violence cannot, of course, be regarded as providing a good sampling ground for real-life violence. Among other differences, there are a number of constraints in the hockey rink that are only replicated in very special subsamples of violent events in other settings. First of all, there are a great many witnesses present in sports, which makes for stricter adherence to rules defining which acts are prescribed, permitted, and proscribed. Implicit rules also determine what resolutions are possible. Another difference from real-life scenarios is that there are designated role carriers with assigned policing functions on the ice (the referee and the linesmen). They will enter the fracas when they judge it strategically advisable or when there seems to be a risk of serious injury to a player. More importantly for our discussion, when challenged, threatened, or provoked, the hockey player does not have available to him the full range of alternatives available in some other contexts. In this regard, the setting to some extent resembles others with spectators present, such as taverns and bars. Unlike the actors in physical combat in other settings, the hockey player cannot try to reason with the adversary, ignore him, or leave the scene (for another part of the rink) without risking being labeled as "chicken," with great carryover for status and identity from one game to the next.

A person's choice of violent acts is determined largely by the context and by the symbolic and interactional meaning of the acts in that context. In an NHL rink, a whole career could be spoiled if a player in a conflict started slapping his adversary instead of engaging in manly fisticuffs and bear hugs. Hair pulling has been executed in one or two memorable fights, to the consternation of spectators, TV commentators, and the TV audience. Kicking would also be out of the question (although it has been observed), and hitting with a weapon (a hockey stick being the most readily available one) is really bending the limits of the permissible. These rules are reflected in the media outrage at some of these occurrences and by the relatively severe penalties meted out to the perpetrators of such violence.

My point is that there are also rules in everyday violence concerning what acts are permitted, even after the boundary of physical violence has been crossed. Rules have their special ranges of applicability; some acts that are permitted in altercations between men are considered unacceptable when directed against a woman. And here we are back at the finding that the gender of the victim determines the nature of acts more than does the gender of the assailant—hardly a good case for natural-frame explanations of violent behavior that exclusively invoke some determinant processes within the organism of the violent person.

ALCOHOL USE AND ACTS OF VIOLENCE

A major aim of the analyses described in this chapter has been to ascertain whether alcohol use (and assessed drunkenness) obliterates or weakens the restrictions applied to physical aggression—an aspect of what has earlier been labeled the "indiscrimination hypothesis."

I have mentioned above that a number of studies have found a positive association between alcohol use and the seriousness of the violent acts committed in violent encounters. These findings rest heavily on records of officially reported violent crimes as kept by the police or courts of justice. Wolfgang (1958) used the number of individual violent acts (e.g., the number of shots, stabs with a knife, etc.) as an indicator of seriousness. He found that homicide events including an excessive number of such acts were more often related to alcohol use than those with fewer violent acts. Tardif (1967) used injuries and type and length of medical care in his assessment of the association between violent crime and alcohol use. He found that the seriousness of violence measured by these postevent consequences was related to the presence of alcohol in the event. On the other hand, Zacker and Bard (1977) found in their study of police calls to family and nonfamily disputes that assaultiveness was not related to alcohol use in such disputes. Moreover, in a Danish study the injuries in sober marital violence were of a more serious nature than when the men concerned had been drinking (Brodersen, Larsen, Bendtsen, Larsen, & Ulrichsen, 1985). With increased methodological stringency, but with more inferential measures, several psychological experiments have shown that more intensive or prolonged electric shocks are administered to (bogus) adversaries when alcohol has been used (e.g., the meta-analyses carried out by Steele and Southwick [1985], and Bushman and Cooper [1990], which include many of these studies).

In addition to the nature of the violent acts, which is examined here in their relationship to alcohol use, the extent to which the violence led to physical injury and to medical consultation and medical care (medication, hospitalization, etc.) can be used as an indicator of the seriousness of violence. All these analyses can be seen as testing specific "severity" or "aggravation" hypotheses regarding the effects of alcohol in aggression. In this section, however, some analyses that are mainly aimed at testing operationalizations of the indiscriminateness notion of alcohol-related violence are presented. This hypothesis states that alcohol use makes the choice of violent acts less dependent on context, setting, and the nature of the target. It is later tested for two victim characteristics: gender and familiarity.

It has been concluded earlier that violent acts are strongly related to the gender of the victimized person. They are also associated with the relationship between the adversaries and the location where the violent episode takes place. Now, is it true that alcohol use is connected with less discriminate use of violence, in the sense that there is less of a difference between the types of violent acts directed at men and at women, and between those directed at persons who are known well to the aggressor (including family members) and at total strangers, when alcohol has been used than when both adversaries are totally sober? We have to remember that the earlier analyses of acts in this chapter have been carried out on the total material of aggressive events (i.e., both alcohol-related and totally sober aggression). Descriptively, everything is in order; the results are, with some reservations and unanswered questions discussed earlier, representative of the populations of most recent events specified through the two-stage sampling procedure. However, in a more explanatory frame, it is also true that some of the relationships found earlier could be affected by alcohol's role in either weakening or strengthening correlations. Also for this reason, it is important to examine separately violent episodes that were preceded by alcohol use and those that were not.

The types of violence to which the victims had been subjected were clearly related to alcohol use prior to the event (Table 7.5). Throwing of objects was about twice as common in sober episodes as it was when alcohol had been used ($\chi^2 = 4.91$, $df = 1$, $p < .05$). Punching ($\chi^2 = 10.33$, $df = 1$, $p < .01$) and kicking ($\chi^2 = 6.36$, $df = 1$, $p < .02$) on the other hand, were more common in violence where either one or both adversaries had been drinking.

Situations in which both adversaries had been drinking differed greatly with regard to settings and types of adversaries from situations in which only the assailant had used alcohol (see Chapter 6, "Patterns of Alcohol Involvement by Assailants and Victims"). The two types of situations may now be compared with regard to acts of violence (Table 7.5). Punching was more common when both had been drinking (although not at a statistically significant level; $\chi^2 = 3.74$, $df = 1$, $p < .10$). Grabbing, pushing, or shoving was more common when only the assailant had consumed alcohol ($\chi^2 = 7.73$, $df = 1$, $p < .01$). The possibility that these differences are explainable by different gender combinations of adversaries, or some other factors related to adversaries or settings in the two types of situations, is examined later.

Compared to the differences found for types of acts separately (Table 7.5), there was little difference in the prevalence of combinations of types of acts between episodes in which the assailant was sober and episodes prior to which the assailant had been drinking. Drinking assailants were more likely to have resorted exclusively to their fists (21% vs. 12%) and less likely to have only slapped their victims (12% vs. 20%).

In violent situations where the assailant was the only drinker, he/she committed more of the listed types of acts—on the average, 1.80 different types of acts, compared to 1.62 when neither had been drinking and a mean of 1.66 when both had been drinking. (It should be noted that "other acts" have been counted as *one* type of act only in these analyses. A few respondents actually listed more than one type of act in this residual category.)

When both the victim and the assailant had been drinking, there was a much higher prevalence of only punching the victim than when only the assailant had used alcohol (26% vs. 16%; $\chi^2 = 3.24$, $df = 1$, $p < .10$). This may reflect the fact that the latter category included more male victims and assailants than the former. Similarly, a 20% prevalence of only grabbing, pushing, or shoving when only the antagonist had been drinking, compared to 9% with both drinking ($\chi^2 = 5.07$, $df = 1$, $p < .05$) could reflect an overrepresentation of female respondents sub-

TABLE 7.5. Violent Acts Committed against the Victim in the Most Recent Episode of Physical Violence, by Various Aspects of Alcohol Involvement

	Hitting with weapon/object	Punching	Kicking	Throwing an object	Slapping	Grabbing pushing, or shoving	Other violent acts
Total ($n = 450$)	15%	43%	20%	12%	36%	36%	7%
Alcohol involved ($n = 225$)	16%	50%	24%	8%	34%	37%	6%
Alcohol not involved ($n = 193$)	16%	34%	14%	16%	41%	33%	7%
Both parties drinking ($n = 114$)	16%	57%	23%	7%	31%	29%	5%
Assailant only drinking ($n = 92$)	15%	44%	26%	10%	35%	48%	5%
Assailant not drinking ($n = 203$)	17%	34%	15%	15%	42%	33%	8%
Assailant drinking ($n = 206$)[a]	16%	51%	24%	8%	33%	38%	5%
Assailant not "drunk" ($n = 59$)	9%	49%	19%	7%	41%	25%	0%
Assailant "drunk" ($n = 128$)	18%	54%	25%	9%	33%	45%	8%
Respondent not drinking ($n = 321$)	15%	37%	18%	13%	37%	38%	8%
Respondent drinking ($n = 114$)	16%	55%	25%	7%	31%	29%	6%
0.5–6.8 cl ($n = 61$)	18%	44%	26%	5%	34%	34%	3%
6.9+ cl ($n = 53$)	13%	68%	25%	9%	26%	23%	9%

[a] *n* for "Assailant drinking" is not equal to the sum of the *n*'s for "Assailant not 'drunk'" and "Assailant 'drunk'" because 19 respondents knew that the assailant had been drinking but could not assess whether he or she was "drunk."

jected to (sexual) harassment by males who had been drinking. (For all other combinations of acts, the distributions were remarkably similar.) A partial test of this possibility—more perspicuous and descriptively meaningful than the more powerful multivariate tests that are described later—is presented in Table 7.6. Punching was more prevalent against victims of both genders when alcohol has been used, but the percentage point difference was greater among men than women (18 compared to 7 points). A finding of greater importance for the indiscrimination hypothesis is that there was actually a greater difference in the prevalence of punching related to the gender of the victim in the alcohol use condition than in the sober condition (38 as compared to 27 percentage points). This act was much less commonly used against female victims in both conditions, and the difference between alcohol-related incidents and sober incidents was statistically significant among male victims ($\chi^2 = 7.87$, $df = 1$, $p < .01$), but not in the victimizations of women. Male victims were kicked much more often in drinking-related incidents ($\chi^2 = 5.81$, $df = 1$, $p < .05$), whereas the difference among female respondents was well within the limits of sampling errors. The gender difference was greater in alcohol-involved incidents here as well (15 as compared to 5 percentage points).

The findings can be summarized as follows: When alcohol was present in violence, there was a somewhat higher likelihood of serious violence (at least punching and kicking) against both men and women. (This support for the severity hypothesis is very weak.) However, the increase over sober violence was greater among male victims. This indicates that *there was in fact a tendency toward more discrimination by gender of the victim, not less, when alcohol had been used.* This finding is

TABLE 7.6. Violent Acts Committed against the Victim in the Most Recent Episode of Physical Violence, as Related to Alcohol Involvement and Gender of Victim

	Male victims		Female victims	
Type of violent act	Alcohol involved ($n = 143$)	No alcohol involved ($n = 102$)	Alcohol involved ($n = 82$)	No alcohol involved ($n = 91$)
Hitting with weapon or object	17%	21%	12%	11%
Punching/hitting with fist	65%	47%	27%	20%
Kicking	30%	17%	15%	12%
Throwing an object	5%	10%	13%	22%
Slapping	23%	33%	52%	51%
Grabbing, pushing, or shoving	29%	25%	51%	42%
Other violent acts	6%	6%	4%	9%

rather tentative, due to the post hoc nature of the methodology. It also needs some further controls, which are instituted later with the help of logistic regression models.

Now let us look at the less serious acts of violence. With these, there was also a tendency toward a greater percentage point difference between men and women in the prevalence of acts when alcohol had been used prior to the violent episode. In sober events, the difference between men and women was 18 percentage points for the act of slapping; when alcohol had been used, it was 29 percentage points (Table 7.6). These patterns again suggest that rather than a tendency toward *less* discrimination based on the gender of victim in alcohol conditions, there was a tendency toward more discrimination.[3] Throwing objects at women was less common in alcohol-related incidents than in sober ones, but this tendency was not statistically significant.

The patterns of violent acts discernible to this point show a tendency toward less difference between alcohol-related and non-alcohol-related acts among female than among male victims. Before this tendency is attributed to the determinant role of alcohol, several competing explanatory possibilities should be considered. One of these is the following: Events in which alcohol was not present might contain a greater proportion of female *assailants*, who would perhaps in part for physical reasons not engage in fisticuffs or kicking the opponent, whether alcohol was present in the situation or not. Table 7.7 shows the patterns of acts as they relate to the combinations of (1) gender of victim and assailant and (2) alcohol use by the assailant. There were not enough female assailants to allow a full breakdown, and thus only events with male assailants have been included.

The table shows that men who had been drinking tended to resort to their fists somewhat more often, regardless of the gender of the target of violence. The most pervasive pattern emerging, however, is the persistence of different types of violence by males if the objects of their violence were women, even when the men had been drinking. There was much more slapping, throwing of objects, and grabbing, pushing, or shoving, as well as much less kicking or punching, against female victims even when the assailants had consumed alcohol. The indiscrimination hypothesis does not receive *any* support from these data. Still, the patterns could no doubt arise from the different relationships typically involved in purely male violent encounters as opposed to those occurring between men and

3. Perhaps this can be conceptualized as more *stereotypical* aggressive behavior after alcohol intake. Whether this will lead onto fertile theoretical ground is an open question at this stage. In the future monograph on subphysical aggression, this characteristic will be deduced from a cognitive theory of alcohol effects.

TABLE 7.7 Violent Acts Committed against the Victim in the Most Recent Episode of Physical Violence, as Related to Alcohol Use by the Assailant and to the Gender of Victims of Male Assailants

	Male assailant–male victim		Male assailant–female victim	
Type of violent act	Assailant drinking ($n = 123$)	Assailant not drinking ($n = 81$)	Assailant drinking ($n = 69$)	Assailant not drinking ($n = 68$)
Hitting with weapon or object	18%	26%	13%	8%
Punching/hitting with fist	68%	53%	29%	18%
Kicking	32%	20%	16%	12%
Throwing an object	5%	10%	15%	21%
Slapping	20%	24%	50%	48%
Grabbing, pushing, or shoving	29%	26%	57%	38%
Other violent acts	6%	6%	3%	10%

women. A final judgment must await the results of regression analyses, since the data do not suffice for further controls by cross-tabular means.

At this point, we can rather safely conclude from the analyses in this section that the effects of alcohol—at least in the amounts consumed by the adversaries in these fairly typical events of physical aggression (and we have to remember that 68% of the assailants who had been drinking were assessed by respondents as having been "drunk")—do not lead to a radical abandonment of the normative strictures regarding what types of violent acts are more permissible than others when a man has a woman as an adversary in physical conflict. To some degree, these differences may be due to the fact that women do not typically put up the same type of resistance as men. However, this would still mean that situational reciprocity rules are not abandoned under the influence of alcohol. These possible interpretations have to await further study for their verification.

Whether the assailant was "drunk" as assessed by the respondent, or had used alcohol but was not considered "drunk," was also related to the choice of violent acts (see Table 7.5 above). Drunken perpetrators had also committed more different types of violence than had other assailants: a mean of 1.92, compared to 1.50 for those who had consumed alcohol but were not drunk, and 1.64 for sober assailants. The only type of act that was more frequent among aggressors who had been drinking but were not considered drunk was slapping the victim. The largest percentage differences in favor of drunken assailants were those for hitting with a weapon or object and grabbing, pushing, or shoving. These differences persisted against both male and female victims (results not shown).

As a final cross-tabular test, a comparison was made between the violent acts committed by male assailants against male and female victims for the cases in which the assailants had not used alcohol and those in which they were judged to be "drunk." The logic of the comparison is parallel to the one exhibited in Table 7.7. However, any tendencies toward indiscriminate violence with increasing alcohol use should be maximally evident in comparing totally sober and obviously intoxicated assailants. Under these two conditions, there were again no remarkable differences for female victims, except for the (by now familiar) greater frequency of grabbing, pushing, or shoving in connection with alcohol use by the assailant: 43% of sober assailants used one or more of these acts, while 60% of drunken assailants did ($\chi^2 = 4.22$, $df = 1$, $p < .05$). This was the only difference among female victims that was significant even on the .05 level. Among men, there were the (also by now familiar) higher rates with alcohol of punching ($\chi^2 = 10.50$, $df = 1$, $p < .01$), kicking ($\chi^2 = 8.30$, $df = 1$, $p < .01$), and grabbing, pushing, and shoving (n.s.); there was also a somewhat lower rate of slapping (n.s.). *The differences between male and female victims in the acts to which they had been subjected were thus actually greater in events in which the assailants were judged to have been "drunk" than when they had not been drinking at all.* Under sober conditions, there was a difference of 26 percentage points in the prevalence of punching victims of different genders; when the assailants were judged to be "drunk," the difference was 43 points. Similarly, the difference for kicking was 4 points when assailants were sober and 27 points when assailants were considered "drunk." Again, these data provide no support for the indiscrimination hypothesis with regard to the gender of the victim.

The amounts of alcohol consumed by the victims themselves before being subjected to violence have been presented with the other alcohol-related measures in Table 7.5. They do not show any clear relationships to the different acts to which the victims were subjected. The differences, as measured in percentage points, between different consumption levels were greatest for punching ($\chi^2 = 6.39$, $df = 1$, $p < .05$), and for grabbing, pushing, or shoving, for which an opposite tendency was evident (n.s.). Slapping also decreased with a higher level of consumption by the victim. Differences between victims who consumed varying amounts may, of course, be explained by the fact that women generally drink smaller amounts of alcohol at one sitting than do men. This further confounding possibility is examined with the help of logistic regression analyses below. It should be pointed out that the cutoff point in Table 7.5 for amounts consumed is not very high—about the equivalent of four bottles of Canadian beer or the same number of 1½-ounce shots of liquor. More distinct patterns may emerge at higher consumption levels.

It should be pointed out that an absence of differences in the violent acts committed in alcohol-involved versus other events does not imply that there may not be a higher risk of the occurrence of *episodes* containing these violent acts when alcohol has been used as compared to when alcohol has not been used. To get at this risk, we would have to sample alcohol use episodes of different kinds and examine how the probability of violence differs from that of a somehow matched sample of events in which alcohol has not been used. This, of course, is easier said than done, although a research strategy of convergent approximations seems possible.

The least that can be said at this point in the current investigation is that alcohol-induced indiscrimination, if the hypothesis is going to survive further tests, will have to be made contingent on other factors than gender of the target of violent acts. These would be factors that have not been controlled for through the collection or handling of the data, and that interact with the use of alcohol (such as certain characteristics of the drinker or the situation) or are related to the alcohol variable itself (such as high threshold levels of consumption before there is any significant increase in the indiscriminate use of aggression and violence). In the application of logistic regression models to the data below, the familiarity of the victim is introduced as another discriminating factor in addition to gender of the victim.

DETERMINANT PATTERNS IN ACTS OF VIOLENCE

The five most common types of violent acts are examined separately in this section. Different sets of characteristics of the adversaries and the setting have been included in logistic regression models, in order to assess their contribution to the likelihood that a specific violent act would be part of a violent encounter. These characteristics are as follows: gender of victim and assailant, age of victim and assailant, extent to which the assailant was known to the victim, and location of the violent incident (i.e., whether it occurred in a private home or elsewhere). In addition to these variables, the influence of drinking by the victim and by the assailant (as well as the latter's assessed drunkenness) has also been examined by means of logistic regression models. Because of the time lag between the occurrence of violence and the interview, factors such as marital status, education, and drinking frequency[4] have not been used in these models.

4. There is some support for the greater relative importance of acute intoxication, which is studied here, than of alcoholic drinking patterns in determining imprisonment for violent crime and arrests for violent crimes during a 12-month period (Collins & Schlenger, 1988). Parallel investigations in general populations are needed.

Some of the models fitted onto the data serve as rough tests of general severity or aggravation hypotheses: (1) Does alcohol use by the assailant increase the likelihood of violence of a more serious nature? (2) Does it increase it more than it increases the probability of milder violent acts? A more direct test of the indiscrimination hypothesis has also been conducted: The incidents have been divided into those in which the assailants had been drinking and those in which the assailants were sober. The extent to which two potentially powerful discriminatory characteristics of the victim—the gender and the closeness of the relationship—influenced the prevalence of different types of acts under the different alcohol conditions is then examined.

First, in a summary fashion, I show the ranked contributions of different factors to the risk of different violent acts. As before in this type of summary, the beta estimates of the different models are not shown, but only their direction and the significance level by which they decrease or increase the probability of the act, and the relative rank of the four most influential variables (Table 7.8).

Slapping the Victim

Slapping was on the average, the least serious type of act, as judged by the extent of injury and medical care sought (no injuries were reported in all 67 cases of mere slapping; see Chapter 8). It is evident that male assailants were less likely than female assailants to slap their victims (Table 7.8). The gender of the victim also determined this behavior, although at lower levels of both determinant strength and confidence in generalizability. (This was the only type of act for which the standardized beta coefficient was not higher, and the determination stronger, for gender of the victim than for gender of the assailant.) Male victims were less likely to be slapped, whether the assailant was a man or a woman.

Assailants who were known very well to their victims (including relatives and family members) were much more likely to slap the victims than were other assailants, independently of the gender constellation. The setting of the conflict also influenced the probability of slapping's being part of the violent episode. Having the conflict in a private home increased the likelihood of this relatively mild type of violent act. Neither drinking by the assailant nor drinking by the victim had any effect whatsoever on the probability that the victim would be slapped when violence occurred.

The assailant's drunkenness was also examined for its impact on slapping as part of violent behavior (not shown in Table 7.8). It neither increased nor decreased the probability of slapping. In order to examine the role of the amount that the victim had imbibed, his/her consumption

TABLE 7.8. Summary of Rank Order, Direction, and Statistical Significance of Risk Factors in Different Logistic Regression Models Determining the Risk That Different Acts of Violence Occur in the Most Recent Episode of Physical Violence

Risk factor	Slapping	Grabbing, pushing, or shoving	Punching	Kicking	Hitting with weapon or object
Male victim	−4**	−1****	+1****	+1	+1
Male assailant	−1***		+2*	+2	
Victim aged under 30		−3*			+2
Assailant aged under 30					−4
Victim knew assailant very well[a]	+2**	−2*	−4		
Incident occurred in a private home	+3**		−3	−4	−3
Victim drinking					
Assailant drinking		+4		+3	

[a]Including relatives and family members.
*$p < .05$.
**$p < .01$.
***$p < .001$.
****$p < .0001$.

at the event was dichotomized at the median (i.e., 6.7 cl of 100% alcohol). This variable had very little effect on the probability that slapping would occur as part of the victimization.

Grabbing, Pushing, or Shoving the Victim

The type of act with the next lowest injury rates when not used in combination with other acts (17%; see Chapter 8) was grabbing, pushing, or shoving. With a very high degree of confidence, it can be asserted that the probability of this type of act decreased when the victim was a man. Conversely, when women were victimized in violence, the probability of grabbing, pushing, or shoving was increased. Earlier, I have speculated that this might be due to a greater risk of violent acts that are in part sexually motivated when women are victimized. On the other hand, we find here that the gender of the assailant had no influence on the probability of this type of act's occurring in violence. This seems contrary to what could be expected if the violence was part of a sexually motivated aggressive advance or attack.

A close relationship between the adversaries decreased the likelihood of grabbing, pushing, or shoving as part of a violent encounter. This is perhaps contrary to expectations, since these acts generally involved a low risk of injury.

More than for any other type of act, drinking by the assailant showed a tendency toward increasing the probability of one or more of these acts of violence (but only at significance levels between .10 and .30 in the different models). The assailant's being drunk strengthened the tendency toward an increased risk of these acts to the .05 level of significance (not shown in the summary presented in Table 7.8). Higher than median consumption by the victim did not have the same effect. I have noted above that assessed intoxication of the assailant did not have at all the same type of influence on the probability of slapping. Thus, this generally more "intimate" type of violent act showed a tendency to increase with drinking, and particularly drinking to the point of apparent intoxication, by the assailant.

Punching the Victim with Fists

Hitting a victim with clenched fists had more serious consequences than the two types of acts hitherto considered; 34% of incidents consisting of mere punching led to injury to the victims (see Chapter 8). Again, neither drinking by the assailant nor drinking by the victim had any significant effect on the likelihood that this type of violence would be used against a victim. The major influence was exerted by the gender of the victim—a pattern that is by now fairly familiar. If the victim was male, the risk of the use of fists increased. An assailant's being male also created a (somewhat weaker) increasing tendency toward the use of fists.

If the violence took place in a private home, and also if the assailant was known very well by the victim, the likelihood of using the fists in violence was somewhat reduced, although not at a statistically significant level. It should perhaps be pointed out that the age of the adversaries, in the dichotomized form employed in this analysis, had no influence on the likelihood of the use of fists in violence. (This may shatter some stereotypes.) Neither drunkenness by the assailant nor relatively high consumption by the victim had a significant effect on the likelihood of use of fists.

Kicking and Hitting with a Weapon or Object

For the two potentially most damaging acts, kicking the victim and hitting him/her with a weapon or object, there were more diffuse determinant patterns. None of the independent variables can be said with standard statistical confidence to have influenced the risk of these two acts. This lack of determination was somewhat clearer for the act of kicking the victim than for hitting with a weapon or object.

Two different types of explanations for this absence of definite patterns come to mind. They are probably linked. According to the first explanation, these types of acts may involve such intense arousal (connected to their serious nature) that discriminatory rules or realistic strategies (e.g., related to the relative strength of the adversaries) are disregarded or completely lose their "inhibitory" meaning. The relative seriousness of the acts is thus an indicator of the state of mind of the assailant. The other, complementary explanation is that no discriminatory rules may exist for these types of actions. They are relatively rare and beyond the permissible in almost all situations, and this may have prevented a set of well-defined and generally agreed-upon discriminatory rules from developing.

Alcohol use by the assailant showed a weak tendency to increase the risk of kicking the victim. Drunkenness by the assailant did not add to the explanatory power over mere drinking by the assailant for either act. Higher than median amounts consumed by the victim did, however, lead to a sizeable increment in the determinant power over mere drinking, but only with regard to hitting the victim with a weapon or object. These tendencies are hard to interpret, and it may be futile to try, since they were not very strong.

Alcohol and the Seriousness and Indiscrimination of Violence

I have noted early on that scientific stereotyping and a powerful explanatory tradition have tended to place alcohol-related violence rather squarely within the frame of natural phenomena. Attention has been focused on direct causal determination by alcohol as a chemical substance and by rather obscurely postulated internal physiological (and some strongly linked psychological) processes that accompany its use. The evidence from the present study shows that this paradigmatic assumption is clearly too one-sided to fit the facts.

In all essential respects, the findings from the cross-tabular analyses have been replicated through logistic regression modeling: Sociodemographic characteristics of the victim were generally more important in determining the violent acts perpetrated than were the same characteristics of the assailant. The significant victim characteristics included gender and closeness of the relationship to the assailant (and, to some extent, age). Among assailant characteristics, only gender was among the four most important determinants with regard to more than one type of violent act. The setting of the violent episode achieved almost the same level of influence. Still, *all* these factors were more important than was alcohol use by either participant.

Alcohol use by the assailant was thus not a major factor in determining the occurrence of any type of violent act in a conflict. There were some weak tendencies for it to increase kicking and grabbing, pushing, or shoving, but no confident generalizations could be made from these analyses. Alcohol use did not tend to increase acts of a more serious nature, such as punching, kicking, and hitting with a weapon or object, any more than it did the two less serious types. The severity hypothesis thus did not receive any support from these data.

What about indiscrimination in aggression as a partial effect of alcohol use? In the cross-tabular analyses presented earlier, it was evident that the indiscrimination hypothesis regarding effects of alcohol did not receive much support from differences between acts to which male and female victims had been subjected. In some analyses, the discrimination between male and female victims in acts to which they had been subjected actually tended to *increase* with alcohol use. Imputed drunkenness, compared to mere drinking by the assailant, did not reveal any additional patterns.

A more direct, although also more specific, test of the indiscrimination hypothesis is carried out here for the purpose of illustrating possible empirical boundaries of the findings and related interpretations regarding alcohol and discrimination up to this point. The relative risks presented in Table 7.9 are based on logistic regression models that were applied to data stratified by whether the assailant had been drinking or not. In order to get away from some potentially confounding interaction effects, only incidents with male assailants have been included in the analyses.

Some rather specific circumstances are used to illustrate the relative risks that a sober and a drinking assailant would use specific types of violent acts. The scenario for which relative risk estimates related to the alcohol use of the assailant are presented in Table 7.9 included the following characteristics: The assailant was a man and the victim was a person over the age of 30.

According to the indiscrimination hypothesis, characteristics of the victim and the setting that under sober conditions would determine what violent acts were committed against a victim would no longer have this effect (or as strong an effect) under the influence of alcohol. Without wishing to imply anything about the types of causal processes potentially involved in bringing about indiscrimination in connection with the use of alcohol, I can also state the hypothesis in the following terms: Characteristics of the setting and the victim that would usually tend to "inhibit" a specific type of act (or the manner of carrying it out) would cease to have this function or effect for an aggressor under the influence of alcohol. (This type of indiscrimination is in fact used to indicate the "disinhibiting," effects of alcohol; even in the theoretical context of alcohol as a "disinhibitor" it is an unnecessarily narrow conception of the determinant processes involved.) In connection with the cross-tabular presentations earlier in the chapter, I have discussed one such factor: the gender of the victim. Another discriminatory characteristic is introduced here: the extent to which the assailant and the victim knew each other. (Other "inhibiting" factors could also be studied, such as the setting of the violence, the presence of witnesses, etc.) The hypothesis as operationalized here thus has the following two corollaries:

1. There should be a smaller risk difference between male and female victims in the assailant's choice of violent acts for an assailant who was drinking, compared to one who was sober.
2. There should be a smaller risk difference between the familiar and less well-known victims in the assailant's choice of violent acts for an assailant who was drinking, compared to one who was sober.

A relative risk value over 1.00 in Table 7.9 means that drinking by a male assailant was associated with a higher risk of the act's being performed against a victim aged 30 and over under the conditions specified to the left of the table. I have mentioned earlier that on the average, drinking assailants committed more different types of acts than did sober

TABLE 7.9. Ratio of Risk That a Violent Act Would Be Carried Out by a Drinking Male Assailant to the Risk That It Would Be Carried Out by a Sober Male Assailant in the Same Type of Situation (All Victims Aged 30 and Over)

	Slapping	Grabbing, pushing, or shoving	Punching	Kicking	Hitting with weapon or object
Male victim who did not know the assailant well	1.18	1.14	1.15	2.24	0.39
Female victim who did not know the assailant well	1.08	1.26	0.78	2.96	0.89
Male victim who knew the assailant well	1.19	2.43	1.26	1.09	0.34

ones. This is in part reflected in the fact that the table shows values greater than 1.00 in 11 out of the 15 cells.

For slapping, the relative risk ratios were almost identical under all three conditions, which implies that there was no indiscrimination for either victim characteristic when a perpetrator had been drinking. For grabbing, pushing, and shoving, there was the same persistence of discrimination based on gender of the victim, while there was a marked increase in this type of violent behavior against a well-known male victim after drinking (2.43 as compared to 1.14 for a less well-known adversary). In other words, for this act there was discrimination with regard to gender of the victim, but indiscrimination with regard to the closeness of the relationship after drinking (at least when a male assailant was facing a male victim). As was also the case for the total sample of victims in the earlier analyses based on simple cross-tabulations, there was actually a *higher* level of discrimination after drinking based on victim's gender for the act of punching (0.78 for a relatively unfamiliar assailant of a woman and 1.15 for a man of low familiarity who victimized another man). No real difference is noticeable for the closeness of male relationships in this regard (1.26 vs. 1.15).

Kicking, by contrast, shows a new pattern: For both unfamiliar male and unfamiliar female victims, there was a much higher than average increase in risk with an assailant's drinking than for the other acts. (This could be seen as supporting the severity hypothesis, but in that case it would be a conditional—in fact, a "discriminating"—support, since the increase was not evident for well-known male victims.) With regard to indiscrimination, there was a tendency for the relative risk to be higher among women, but the difference is not great enough to base generalizations on. A comparison between the well-known and less well-known male victims (1.09 vs. 2.24) actually shows *more* discrimination after drinking, since strangers and near-strangers were the ones kicked disproportionately often after drinking. Lastly, hitting with a weapon or object shows values well under unity (at least for the group of assailants and victims used in this illustration). There was less discrimination based on gender of victim (0.89 for females, compared to 0.39 for males), but since the severity was clearly reduced with drinking assailants, it is hard to interpret this as mere indiscrimination. Familiarity of male victims did not cause any difference in relative risk; the figures are practically identical (0.39 and 0.34).

Some of the findings shown in Table 7.9 are no doubt specific to the groups selected for the illustration. What remains is a rather complicated pattern that definitely does not lend any unconditional support to a general indiscrimination hypothesis. Different patterns seem to emerge with regard to different discriminatory variables. No interaction effects have been examined because of the relatively modest sample sizes. Replications with larger samples of violent incidents, in which interaction effects can be systematically studied, are needed. So are experimental models for replicative purposes.

The next chapter addresses the question of whether indiscrimination is reflected more unambiguously in the *injuries* sustained by the victims. The interpretations pertaining to injuries are simpler, since we are only dealing with one dependent variable and do not have to take into account a whole pattern of such variables, as in the examination of the different types of violent acts. However, it is clear from both the cross-tabulations and the regression analyses presented here that different kinds of acts are predominantly used against women and against men. This is true both when the assailants are sober and when they have used alcohol prior to the conflict. It is reflected in the following news item, describing an incident in which all participants had been drinking:

> The married couple went to a restaurant to enjoy an evening of love and good will. However, the evening ended with the 40-year-old husband hitting both his wife and a mutual male acquaintance.
>
> During the festive meal the wife went to the restroom. After a while the mutual acquaintance also disappeared from the table. He also said that he was going to visit the restroom.
>
> However, it took a long time before the wife and the good friend returned, and the husband was getting suspicious. He went to the ladies' room, but his wife was not there. Now the husband started getting seriously alarmed. He broke open the door to the men's room.
>
> Both his wife and the mutual acquaintance were standing there without their pants on. The jilted husband was enraged. He hit both his wife and the man, the wife with an open hand and the man with a clenched fist. (*Expressen*, Stockholm, Sweden, April 27, 1988; my translation)

8

Injuries Incurred and Medical Care Sought as a Result of Violence

We all know that some violence has extremely serious consequences. Permanent or long-term damage can be done to close relationships, to mental and physical health, to personal and family finances, and to many other aspects of existence seriously affecting a person's whole life. Often the victim pays a higher price than the assailant, even when relief, restitution, or plain physical security is sought and gained by legal or other means:

"I didn't know my husband was on speed until afterwards. . . . The beatings happened almost every night. He was drinking a lot, too. Some nights he didn't come home. I got a lawyer and had a separation, and he was evicted from our home. Then we had a divorce. I had the children out for adoption to protect them from him getting them."

"My husband kept me prisoner at home. When I went out he shot me. I was taken to hospital in an ambulance."

The respondents were asked to describe in an open-ended fashion how and why the most recent episode of violence ended (see question 11 in Appendix B). In about 12% of the cases, the violence ended in physical incapacitation of the victim or the assailant ("passing out," being pinned down on the floor, etc). References to incapacitation and fights were much more common in all-male encounters; such terminations of the conflict were cited in 32% of all-male violent episodes. When at least one of the adversaries was female, they were referred to in only 10% of cases. Another 10% of the victims described the end of the conflict in such terms as "It petered out," mainly through some interactional dynamics (without incapacitation in any form); a further 20% ascribed it mainly to intervention by the police and others. In 19% of the incidents, passive acceptance of the violence (including attempts at reasoning with the assailant) was seen as having a predominant role in ending the violence. In another 15%, closure of the episode was achieved (in the view of the respondent) in a relatively friendly manner, such as with handshakes, apologies, tears, hugs and kisses, and the like. The two last-mentioned endings to the aggressive interaction (passive acceptance and friendliness) were more common when at least one woman was involved. In another 18% the victim or assailant left the scene of his/her own accord—in some cases fleeing, in other cases just walking away (before any of the other resolutions had a chance to develop). Finally, a remaining 6% of victimized respondents cited the end of violence in terms that were not classifiable in the above categories.

INJURIES AND MEDICAL CARE AS RELATED TO DIFFERENT TYPES OF VIOLENT ACTS

Respondents were asked a straightforward question on whether they had been injured in their most recent victimization: "Were you injured at all?" (question 19, Appendix B). This left it up to each respondent to define physical injury. More serious injuries led a victim to seek medical care or medical advice; in other cases self-medication was felt to be sufficient. The respondents were asked whether they, as a result of their injuries, had sought medical help ("What did you do about [your injury]? Did you go to a hospital, doctor, or nurse?"—question 20a, Appendix B) and whether they had taken (internally) or applied (externally) any medication ("Did you take or apply any medication?"—question 20b, Appendix B). In some cases, the victim did both.

Out of the 435 respondents (unweighted figure) who reported on their most recent victimization by physical violence, 26% reported having been physically injured. A hospital, doctor, or nurse was contacted in 11% of the cases, and an equal proportion of victims reported having used or applied some kind of medication.

One would, of course, expect a relationship between the type of acts to which a victim is subjected and the risk of injury. Episodes that included hitting with a weapon or an object, and those including punching, kicking, and throwing of objects at the victim, had very similar injury rates (about 40%). However, the "other violent acts" category (i.e., incidents consisting of acts of violence other than those listed to the respondent) tended to have a higher probability of injury than incidents in which listed types of acts occurred (57%). In addition to the high proportion of injuries in such incidents, these miscellaneous violent acts also led the victims to seek medical care and to use medication to a greater extent than in other violent incidents.

These results pertain to episodes in which other types of acts in addition to the designated ones may have been directed at the victim; they refer, for instance, to episodes of physical violence in which *at least* kicking occurred. (As I have noted in Chapter 7, there was a mean of 1.68 different types of violent acts per incident; 63% of the incidents included only one type of act, 21% two types of acts, and 17% three or more types of acts.) For the four most common single-type episodes (the ones with enough cases to allow at least tentative estimates), the following prevalences of injuries were obtained:

Only slapping: 0% ($n = 67$)
Only grabbing, pushing, or shoving: 17% ($n = 60$)
Only kicking: 27% ($n = 22$)
Only punching: 34% ($n = 76$)

The reason why punching caused at least as much injury as kicking is probably related to the fact that punching is disproportionately aimed at the head and particularly the face—an area that is both vulnerable and visible. The face is the major locus for emotional expression and the transmission of messages and signs. Its role as the main objectively available site of the social and interactional self probably explains the concentration of violence in this area of the human body.

Reversing the base (see Table 8.1) has revealed the prevalence of the different acts used against the respondents in injury events and events that led to medical activity—a useful exercise, since it has provided the *type* of sample used in analyzing health care and emergency room cases (although injuries treated in emergency rooms are typically more serious). In the table, a comparison is made with violence episodes that fell outside this type of sampling frame—violence in which no injuries were sustained. There were marked differences in types of acts committed between episodes that led to injury (and medical activity) and those in which the victim was not hurt physically.

With the exception of slapping, there was a distinct overrepresentation of all different types of acts in injury events. Grabbing, pushing, or shoving was at the null hypothesis level. The general overrepresentation was related to the fact that the mean number of different types of acts was 2.10 in episodes that resulted in injury to the respondent, compared to the

TABLE 8.1. Violent Acts Committed in Most Recent Episode of Physical Violence, as Related to Victim's Injury and Medical Activity

Type of violent act	No injury to victim ($n = 331$)	Victim injured ($n = 119$)	Victim sought medical help ($n = 48$)[a]	Victim used medication ($n = 48$)[a]
Hitting with weapon or object	12%	24%	33%	33%
Punching/hitting with fist	36%	62%	67%	69%
Kicking	16%	30%	29%	26%
Throwing an object	9%	17%	21%	19%
Slapping	40%	26%	31%	23%
Grabbing, pushing, or shoving	36%	36%	40%	38%
Other violent acts	4%	15%	23%	19%

[a]These were subsamples of the "victim injured" sample, and also overlapped between themselves. Thus the distributions of the last three columns are not independent of one another.

overall mean of 1.68. The corresponding mean numbers of types of acts for medical consultation and medication events were 2.44 and 2.25, respectively. The higher number of acts in incidents that led to physical injury and medical activity may indicate that there was more escalation from mild to severe violent acts and/or a greater proportion of violent encounters that could be characterized as "brawls" in incidents that led to injury. Events with a greater number of types of violence were probably also disproportionately extended in time.

Combinations of acts (especially combinations of three or more types of acts) were more common in incidents with injury to the victim—35% as compared to 19% in episodes in which the victim was not injured ($\chi^2 = 12.22$, $df = 1$, $p < .001$). Incidents in which the respondent was only punched were also overrepresented in injury cases—22% versus 16% (n.s.). On the other hand, mere grabbing, pushing, or shoving, and especially slapping, were underrepresented among episodes resulting in injury.

Violence in which there was injury to the victim, and especially violence that was serious enough to lead to medical activity, could be expected to lead to a greater proportion of police attention. This has been borne out by the facts (Table 8.2). Clearly, injury to the victim, especially of the kind that led him/her to seek the care of medical personnel, was very important in determining police involvement and court charges. Fully 33% of incidents where the victim was injured and 44% of cases where he/she sought professional medical care for the injuries came to the attention of the police. This should be compared to the overall mean of 15%.

TABLE 8.2. Sociolegal Consequences of the Most Recent Episode of Physical Violence, as Related to the Victim's Injuries and Medical Activity

	Police involved	Charges laid
No injury to victim (n = 119)	8%	3%
Victim injured (n = 332)	33%	11%
No contact with hospital, doctor, or nurse by the victim (n = 402)	11%	3%
Victim contacted hospital, doctor, or nurse (n = 48)	44%	20%
No use of medication by the victim (n = 401)	12%	4%
Victim used medication (n = 48)	28%	19%

INJURIES AND MEDICAL ACTIVITY AS RELATED TO PARTICIPANTS AND SETTINGS

Gender-Related Findings

Medical activity rates followed injury rates across a number of different situational and background variables. From the fact that generally more severe acts were committed when men rather than women were subjected to violence (Table 7.1), it could be predicted that men would report getting injured in a greater share of their victimizations than women. This has been borne out in the summary of findings shown in Table 8.3, although the difference was not great: 29% of men reported that they were physically injured, compared to 22% of women. Men were also more likely to seek medical help or to use some medication, especially the latter, both independently and in conjunction with each other.

A comparison revealed no great differences for either male or female victims in injury rates and medical activity between the total sample of violent events and those that occurred within city limits during an 8-year period immediately preceding the interview. In the latter subsample, 27% of male victims were injured (compared to 29% in the total sample). For female victims, the corresponding figures were 19% and 22%. Contacts with medical caregivers occurred in identical proportions, while medication was used in 9% of the more recent occurrences in the city (compared to 11% for the total sample). There were thus very weak indications that the more recent episodes reported were of a somewhat milder nature than the older ones. This may have been an outcome of faulty recall: The less serious episodes further back in time may have been forgotten, and relatively serious ones may have been reported instead. However, the tendency was very weak and did not affect the findings to any relevant degree.

TABLE 8.3. Injuries and Medical Activity in the Most Recent Episode of Physical Violence, as Related to Characteristics of the Assailant, Victim, and Setting

	Victim was injured	Victim contacted hospital, doctor, nurse	Victim used some medication
Total ($n = 451$)	26.4%	10.8%	10.8%
Gender of victim			
Male ($n = 270$)	29%	13%	14%
Female ($n = 181$)	22%	8%	6%
Gender of assailant			
Male ($n = 377$)	28%	12%	12%
With male victim ($n = 232$)	33%	15%	15%
With female victim ($n = 143$)	21%	8%	6%
Female ($n = 74$)	19%	6%	7%
Age of assailant			
15–19 ($n = 104$)	27%	7%	13%
20–29 ($n = 180$)	25%	11%	10%
30–39 ($n = 74$)	31%	11%	11%
40 and over ($n = 91$)	24%	16%	11%
Age of victim			
15–19 ($n = 107$)	28%	11%	14%
20–29 ($n = 172$)	24%	9%	9%
30–39 ($n = 78$)	23%	9%	7%
40 and over ($n = 91$)	36%	18%	14%
Location of incident			
Own home ($n = 155$)	17%	7%	7%
Other private home ($n = 47$)	22%	13%	11%
Work or school ($n = 68$)	26%	9%	8%
Public drinking place ($n = 74$)	32%	12%	11%
Street, park, etc. ($n = 62$)	38%	12%	16%
Some other place ($n = 40$)	44%	21%	21%
Relationship of assailant to victim			
Spouse ($n = 92$)	21%	11%	10%
Other family member or relative ($n = 51$)	12%	2%	5%
Extent to which victim knew unrelated assailant			
Very well or fairly well ($n = 134$)	14%	5%	6%
Only a little or hardly at all ($n = 72$)	36%	15%	17%
Not at all ($n = 121$)	41%	16%	13%

Forty-two percent of men who were injured ($n = 79$) and 35% of injured women ($n = 40$) sought medical help from a hospital, doctor, or nurse. This may be a sign that there were no great differences in males' and females' definitions of "injury," although this is a matter that deserves more detailed study.

Male assailants caused injury in 28% of the incidents (Table 8.3), a somewhat higher share than the proportion of community residents injured after being victimized by a female adversary, 19% (n.s.). Medical activity rates followed the same pattern.

Gender of victim and assailant thus influenced the rates of injury and remedial activity. The analyses described in Chapter 7 also showed that the gender combination of interactants in violence was related to the type of acts committed in the course of the violence. From this, one might expect that the gender constellation would show a relationship with the consequences of violence. Table 8.3 shows that violent episodes involving only males led to a much higher proportion of injuries (33%) and medical activity than those with a male assailant and female victim (21% injured). The difference is significant on the .05 level ($\chi^2 = 5.88$, $df = 1$). The medical activity rates for the victims in incidents with only male participants were about double those when a man subjected a woman to violence. (This finding may to some extent reflect women's reluctance to seek help for injuries sustained in domestic violence. Related to this is the fact that when women seek medical care, they tend to blame injuries from domestic violence on accidents; e.g., see Hedeboe et al., 1985; Malterud, 1982.)

The combination of a man as assailant and a woman as the victim did not differ appreciably in any of the three consequences from incidents in which the assailant was a woman. This finding may represent another instance of the fact that acts of violence (in common with other types of interaction) are influenced more by the constellation of interactants, setting, and other factors than by the characteristics of the attacker alone. One discriminating characteristic in everyday violence is the presence of a female participant; this, together with reciprocity norms, determines what is permissible, what the signs are of going too far, when the violent interaction has reached a commonly "acceptable" resolution, and the like. Battering a woman is usually a no-win game for shared everyday definitions of status and identity: It is not seen as a fair fight. Thus there is no winner by the criteria applied by society and significant others. Very strict, graded, and rather finely calibrated rules are usually found for intergender aggression and violence. If an acceptable threshold is crossed, the point of the violence has to be defined in other terms than domination or victory. Often this conceptualization is grounded in a purported natural frame (e.g., "I was drunk") and also uses expressions derived from it ("I was under a great deal of stress," "I just blew up when she . . ."). (Within other definitional paradigms that are totally inappropriate for defining social status or socially acceptable identity, such as a sadistic paradigm of omnipotent power, a satisfactory definition can be achieved even in such situations, and no natural-frame rationalizations are usually made.) When social strictures are abandoned or never existed, both the social and psychodynamic "meaning" of violence changes. Such cases are overrepresented in emergency rooms and in the official records of the police and the courts.

Findings Related to Age and Location

The prevalence of reported injury to the victim did not appear to have any strong or clear-cut relationship to the age of the assailant or the age of the victim (Table 8.3). Injuries were more common in the oldest victim group (who were also subjected to more serious acts). Among victims aged 40 or over, there was also an increase in medical care sought for injuries, but the differences were not statistically significant. Medication use was even less closely related to age of victim or assailant.

Violence in the home of the victim had the lowest rates of injury and of medical action taken (Table 8.3). Streets and parks, and miscellaneous locations, had the highest rates of injury. The latter also seemed to contain the most serious types of injuries, judging from the high levels of medical action. Public drinking places fell into the middle range in both injuries and injury-related curative action. There was no significant difference between men and women in the prevalence of injuries sustained in their own homes (20% and 16%, respectively) or in medical action taken.

Findings Related to the Relationship between Adversaries

Injuries were slightly less common in marital violence than in violence generally, but still one-fifth of violence between spouses led to physical injury to the victim (Table 8.3). The levels of medical activity did not differ from the mean values for the total sample of episodes. However, divorced or separated individuals had the highest rates of injury and of medical care (41% and 24%, respectively; $n = 37$), which again suggests the seriousness of marital violence in problem marriages (these figures are not shown in the table). Recalculations from the 1982 Canadian Urban Victimization Survey indicate that about 13% of female victimizations by males were perpetrated by spouses or ex-spouses. Fully 61% of these led to physical injury in the women, while 24% of assaults by other men did (Solicitor General, Canada, 1985a). (The authors of the 1982 survey suggest that domestic incidents may have been more likely to be reported in the telephone interviews when they led to injury, while the threshold for reporting other male assaults may have been lower, and the injury rates consequently also lower.) These high proportions were connected with higher percentages found for medical treatment, compared to those in the present study: Close to 17% of female assault victims of male aggressors received medical treatment, compared to the present figure of 8%. The lower criteria set for physical violence in the present study no doubt explain a major part of the difference.

In this study, the lowest levels of injury were found among those victims who had been subjected to violence by a family member other than a spouse or by a relative. Strangers and near-strangers caused more injuries than any other group. In keeping with this, the proportion of victims who sought medical help or took or applied medication was also higher in violence between strangers (Table 8.3).

Restricting the present analyses to incidents involving assailants who were not members of the victims' families or otherwise related to them could to some extent control for the fact that women tended to be involved more in violence with family members and relatives. This could explain both the finding that women received fewer injuries and the finding that injuries in intimate and near-intimate relationships were less common than in other relationships. To test this possibility, violence between nonfamily members and nonrelatives was divided into those cases in which the assailant was known to the victim at least to some degree and those in which the assailant was a total stranger. Through this procedure, the sample sizes for female victims became relatively small (largely due to the fact that a substantial proportion of women were last victimized by the spouse or another family member or relative). However, differences in injury rates still achieved admissible levels of statistical significance.

Both women and men were victimized more seriously when the assailant was a total stranger. The percentage differences were considerably greater among women; 16% were injured when the nonrelated assailant was known at least a little, compared to 46% in victimizations by total strangers ($\chi^2 = 8.50$, $df = 1$, $p < .01$). However, the difference among men (25% compared to 39%) also reached a statistically significant level ($\chi^2 = 4.60$, $df = 1$, $p < .05$). In keeping with these findings, medical activity rates were consistently higher when the assailant was a total stranger, and more pronouncedly so among women. The multivariate roles of gender and relationship between antagonists in determining risk of injury are discussed later when the findings from logistic regression analyses are presented.

Is it the choice of acts or the way in which they are executed (the force used, the number of acts, the part of the body assaulted, etc.) that causes strangers to inflict more harm? We have seen earlier that strangers tended to use acts of a more dangerous nature (Table 7.1). From Table 8.4, it is evident that the same acts may also have been carried out more vehemently by strangers. Injury rates were higher in violence between strangers with all three types of acts. Rates of remedial activity were also generally higher in such incidents, although the differences were not great by any means. The only statistically significant difference in injury rates was that for hitting with a weapon or object (23% vs. 57%; $\chi^2 = 6.12$, $df = 1$, $p < .05$). Judging by the high level of medical care in incidents where a weapon or object was used against the victim, it would seem that the choice and/or use of a weapon was more savage in violent conflict between strangers. It is also possible that there was more general use of more than one type of serious acts between strangers, and that this would to some extent account for the differences found. Descriptively, the findings still retain their relevance.

Only the three potentially most dangerous types of acts have been included in the analyses of Table 8.4, since the effects of milder violence (such as slapping) would in many cases be more seriously confounded with other acts used by the assailant in the same incident. (For incidents including slapping, the difference in injury rates was also great between episodes with known assailants and total strangers: 11% vs. 44%. For grabbing, pushing, or shoving, the respective shares were 18% and 39%. Differences in medical activity rates were proportionately even greater. All this may indicate a greater likelihood of escalation in violence between strangers—an interesting question for further study.)

Findings Related to Number of Assailants and Role of Witnesses

In 14% of the violent incidents, more than one person committed some act of violence against the victim. These occasions were related to a dramatically higher risk of injury and remedial activity (Table 8.5). Over half of victims of more than one assailant (57%) were injured, compared to about one-fifth (21%) of those who only had one assailant ($\chi^2 = 35.68$, $df = 1$, $p < .001$). The victims' medical activity followed the same pattern, with about a threefold increase in this prevalence for multiple-assailant incidents over the incidents with only one assailant. These differences also surpassed the .001 level of significance (with χ^2 values of 11.52 and 19.95 for medical contacts and medication, respectively).

At least one person who did not (originally) participate in the violence observed the episode in 66% of the cases. In 43% of these, one or more witnesses tried to prevent the violence from erupting or attempted to stop it once it had started. Table 8.5 shows the relationship between the

TABLE 8.4. Injuries and Medical Activity in the Most Recent Episode of Physical Violence, as Related to Types of Acts used by Assailants Who Were Known to Their Victims and by Total Strangers

	Hitting with weapon/object		Punching		Kicking	
	Known ($n = 30$)	Stranger ($n = 21$)	Known ($n = 90$)	Stranger ($n = 69$)	Known ($n = 41$)	Stranger ($n = 33$)
Victim injured	23%	57%	31%	45%	29%	42%
Victim contacted hospital, doctor, or nurse	17%	43%	12%	19%	12%	12%
Victim took or applied medication	20%	38%	14%	16%	12%	15%

TABLE 8.5. Injuries and Medical Activity in the Most Recent Episode of Physical Violence, as Related to Number of Assailants, Presence of Witnesses, and Intervention by Witnesses

	Victim was injured	Victim contacted hospital, doctor, nurse	Victim used some medication
Total ($n = 451$)	26.4%	10.8%	10.8%
Number of assailants			
One ($n = 386$)	21%	9%	8%
More than one ($n = 64$)	57%	24%	27%
Number of witnesses present			
None ($n = 149$)	18%	7%	9%
1–2 ($n = 100$)	29%	13%	12%
3–9 ($n = 97$)	26%	15%	12%
10 or more ($n = 96$)	35%	10%	24%
Intervention by witnesses ($n = 291$)			
Tried to stop violence ($n = 124$)	31%	15%	14%
Did not try to stop violence ($n = 167$)	30%	11%	10%

presence and role of these other people and injury and medical activity. There was a rather clear cutoff point with regard to both injury and medical activity between violent events with no witnesses and those with at least one person witnessing the violence. Thirty percent of violent incidents witnessed by other people led to injury, by contrast with 18% of totally private violent incidents. The difference in injury rates was significant on the .01 level ($\chi^2 = 7.32$), and the differences in both types of medical activity were significant on the .05 level ($\chi^2 = 4.02$ and 4.47, respectively). There was no significant or systematic difference between occasions with differing numbers of witnesses (with the exception of the much more common use of medication in occasions with 10 or more witnesses, which seems difficult to explain in a nomothetic manner).

In incidents with at least one witness, there was practically no difference in injury or medical activity between occasions in which someone tried to stop the violence and those in which no one made any attempt to stop it. This may be an indication that witnesses will "allow" violence to get to a certain point, but if there are signs that this threshold is surpassed (and the violence "gets out of hand" or may result in serious injury), they will step in and try to prevent further violence. The lack of difference in injury rates would then also indicate that intervention by others may come too late and fail to prevent injury, compared to public violence in which the resolution is left up to the participating individuals.

There may be more apprehension felt by, and an objectively higher risk of injury to, a peacemaker in entering a conflict that has already developed into serious violence. In the following incident described in the "Letters to the Editor" section of a Swedish newspaper, the implication is that the seriousness of injury in this alcohol-related episode could have been reduced by more prompt intervention:

> It was Friday. Three days before Christmas Eve. My friend Jens, who had just returned home from a 3-year stay abroad, and I were going out for a night on the town. He was curious about "Stockholm by night." . . .
>
> What do you do at a disco? Well, you dance, hope to meet a nice old friend or maybe even a nice girl. After all, you are a bachelor. And forget the Christmas stress, the job, unwashed dishes, bills, and everything else for 2 or 3 hours. That's what I thought, anyway. Suddenly, as I stood on the dance floor, three men came forth. They started pushing me and provoking me. "What the hell are you doing?" I asked one of them.
>
> "What! Are you looking for trouble, boy?!"
>
> "Lay off it, and don't be childish."
>
> Pow!
>
> I felt the taste of blood in my mouth.
>
> "What are you doing? Lay off it!" I told them.
>
> Pow! Pow! Pow! Pow!
>
> By now the blood was running from both my nose and my mouth.
>
> "Do you feel better now?" I asked.
>
> Pow! Pow!
>
> Now, I was also fighting ferociously, until one of the bouncers finally woke up. My feelings were mixed when I returned to the fresh air outside to cool down for a while. I was just about to return inside, [but then] what did I see? Outside the disco stood Jens, surrounded by the [first] three guys plus another three. The bouncers outside just stood there watching the melee. I walked over to them and asked them to stop it.
>
> "There are six of you and I'm sure that you can beat us. But what do you gain by doing that? Please, leave us alone." . . . Pow!
>
> The result: One shoe hit my chin. . . . Two and a half hours at the dental surgeon. Two fractures in my chinbone. Adjustment of the chin, which means that my upper teeth and my lower teeth are wired together and that I can only have liquid food for a month. Goodbye to all the Christmas ham, sausages, head cheese. . . .
>
> If one of you guys who were involved that night [should] read this: Booze it up as much as you want to, and fight with those who want to fight. But leave those who do not booze and brawl alone.
>
> Last but not least, I want to thank the bouncers for their outstanding contribution. What in heaven's name were they there for?—Johnny Bryggman (*Dagens Nyheter*, Stockholm, Sweden, December 31, 1984; my translation)

RELATIONSHIPS OF ALCOHOL USE TO INJURIES AND MEDICAL ACTIVITY

From the severity hypothesis, we might expect injuries to be more frequent and serious, and resulting medical activity to be more common, with increasing alcohol involvement. I have already referred to the literature, which points to a greater vehemence in violent episodes where alcohol was involved, although contrary findings have also been reported. In the present data, however, there was hardly any difference in the rate of injury between incidents in which alcohol was involved (27%) and those in which it was not (24%). These results are shown in Table 8.6. This absence of generalizable differences was evident for both male and female victims.

The risk of injury increased with the amount consumed by the victim (Table 8.6), however. In the highest consumption category (more than 10.2 cl of 100% alcohol), about half the respondents reported getting injured and one-fourth reported seeking medical assistance. The difference in injury rates between respondents who had consumed different amounts of alcohol was significant on the .01 level ($\chi^2 = 9.26$, $df = 2$). This finding receives inferential support from several studies of victims of homicide and other violence. These regularly show blood alcohol concentration (BAC) levels considerably above what could be expected from mean amounts consumed by the respondents on their most recent drinking occasions and by the victims of violence (and threats) in the present study.

For instance, Goodman et al. (1986) found that 30% of the homicide victims in the city of Los Angeles had a BAC of 0.10% or more (i.e., 65% of victims who had consumed alcohol), and 13.5% (29% of drinking victims) had a level of at least 0.20%. Cherpitel (1989) found that 30% of patients presenting at an emergency room in San Francisco with injuries from fights or assaults had BACs of at least 0.10%. These patients accounted for 68% of all alcohol-positive cases. The mean BAC in victims of homicide studied by Westermeyer and Brantner (1972) was 0.177%. Dahl, Wickström, and Bo (1981) found that 26 out of 40 alcohol-positive victims of violence accepted for hospital care in Stavanger, Norway had a BAC of at least 0.15%. In Denmark, Möller-Madsen et al. (1986) found that 51% of victims of violence with positive blood alcohol tests who sought medical care at hospital casualty departments had BACs of at least 0.15% ($n = 488$). In Finland, Virkkunen's (1974) study showed a mean BAC of 0.25% in alcohol-related victim-precipitated homicides, and 0.21% in other homicides. These levels are also much higher than the ones used in experimental studies of alcohol's effects on aggression,

TABLE 8.6. Injuries and Medical Activity in the Most Recent Episode of Physical Violence, as Related to Various Characteristics of Alcohol Involvement

	Victim was injured	Victim contacted hospital, doctor, nurse	Victim used some medication
Total ($n = 450$)	26%	11%	11%
No alcohol involved ($n = 199$)	24%	8%	11%
Male victim ($n = 108$)	27%	11%	14%
Female victim ($n = 91$)	21%	4%	8%
Alcohol involved ($n = 226$)	27%	12%	10%
Male victim ($n = 144$)	32%	14%	14%
Female victim ($n = 82$)	20%	10%	3%
Respondent not drinking ($n = 317$)	26%	10%	11%
Respondent drinking ($n = 132$)	29%	13%	11%
Less than 3.5 cl ($n = 26$)	20%	12%	12%
3.5–10.2 cl ($n = 59$)	24%	12%	14%
More than 10.2 cl ($n = 29$)	52%	24%	10%
Assailant not drinking ($n = 208$)	23%	8%	11%
Assailant drinking ($n = 209$)	27%	12%	10%
Not "drunk" ($n = 78$)	25%	11%	13%
"Drunk" ($n = 129$)	27%	14%	9%
Both drinking ($n = 114$)	26%	13%	11%
Assailant only drinking ($n = 92$)	26%	11%	8%

where a BAC of 0.11% is considered too great for most experimental objectives, resulting as it does in total drunkenness (Jones & Vega, 1972).

Studies of prolonged heavy drinking with resulting extreme BACs and often highly irrational behavior tend to have a case study format, and there are no systematic findings related to length of time under the influence and BAC levels in binges that result in serious violent crimes. With the changes in drug use habits of especially high-risk populations during the last 20 years, it has also become increasingly difficult to distinguish drug from alcohol effects (see, e.g., Senay & Wettstein, 1983).

In the present data, there was a sizeable difference in mean consumption between the victims who reported physical injury and those who did not. In incidents in which drinking respondents were injured, their mean consumption was 13.1 cl of 100% alcohol ($n = 34$), compared to 7.4 cl in the incidents in which respondents were not injured ($n = 81$). These amounts correspond to about 12 and 7 ounces of distilled spirits or 8 and 4½ bottles of Canadian beer, respectively.

Drinking by the victim was not differentially associated with either type of medical activity. Victims who resorted to at least one of the two types of medical action as a result their injuries had consumed a mean of 13.3 cl of absolute alcohol ($n = 21$), compared to 12 cl ($n = 13$) for those who were injured but did not take any medical action. There was no generalizable difference, in other words.

When the assailant had been drinking, 27% of victims reported getting injured, as compared to 23% when the assailant had not consumed alcohol (Table 8.6). The differences with regard to medical activity were not of any theoretical or practical significance, either.

Taking the injured victims as a base for calculating rates of medical care provided only small samples to work with but showed some relevant tendencies. The data lend very weak support to a conditional severity hypothesis. When the assailant had not been drinking, 36% of injured respondents ($n = 47$) sought medical care; when he/she had been drinking, 46% of those injured ($n = 57$) did so (n.s.). When the assailant was judged to be "drunk," half of injury cases sought medical care ($n = 36$), leaving the rate for drinking but not drunk antagonists at about the level for sober assailants who caused injuries (38%; $n = 21$). The rates for taking or applying medication showed weak opposing tendencies, and thereby weaken the case for alcohol-induced aggravation in "everyday" violence.

If we are to judge by the results of Table 8.6, the amounts of alcohol consumed by victims were related to injury rates, but this did not seem to be the case for the degree of intoxication of assailants. This finding could be a partial consequence of the general unreliability of the "measure" of drunkenness for assailants; it was not possible to assess gradations of consumption and intoxication for assailants in the same way as for victims. It should also be recalled that the increases in injuries and in seeking of medical care were only noticeable in the highest consumption category of the victims.

In violence where both adversaries had been drinking, the injury rate was the same as when only the assailant had been drinking (Table 8.6). Neither form of medical activity was significantly related to these two types of alcohol involvement.

In order to control for the gender of the assailant as well as the gender of the victim, the results related to drinking by the assailant have been examined for male and female victims of only male assailants (Table 8.7). In all-male encounters, there were hardly any differences on the indicators of seriousness of violence between incidents in which the assailant had been drinking and those in which he had not. Male victims showed elevated levels over female victims on all three dependent factors, whether the assailant had been drinking or not. Here the data provide some (albeit, considering the lack of statistical significance, very weak) support for the indiscrimination hypothesis: Injury rates between the male and female victims of male assailants differed less when the assailants had been drinking (10 percentage points) than when they had not been drinking (15 percentage points). With regard to medical consultation, the tendency was in the same direction (3 as compared to 12 percentage points). There was no tendency in either direction with regard to self-medication (a difference of 11 points for both conditions). The severity hypothesis does not receive any conditional support from this analysis, since injury and medical activity were not related to drinking by the assailant for either male or female victims. The only tendency in this direction was found in care seeking among female victims.

Up to this point, we have seen that the gender constellation of assailant and victim explains injury and medical activity rates to a greater extent than does drinking by the assailant. We also have seen again that there is little or no support for either alcohol-induced severity or indiscrimination related to gender of the victim. However, the best way of assessing the relative contributions of the constellation of participant characteristics and alcohol use by participants (and a good complement to cross-tabular perspicuity) is a more powerful multivariate method. The results of logistic regression analyses with injury to the victim as a dependent variable are studied later. First let us look at another factor besides gender of the victim along which discrimination can be expected, and which should be reflected in variations in rates of injury.

I have noted in Chapter 6 that alcohol was involved more in violent encounters with strangers than in violence with assailants who were to some extent known by the victim. I have also noted earlier in this chapter that the same acts of violence were more likely to be associated with injuries when violence occurred between strangers (Table 8.4). The characteristics linked to alcohol involvement may therefore in part be caused by the fact that alcohol-involved violence is disproportionately made up of violence between strangers. For this reason, it is worthwhile to study the question of whether degree of intimacy and alcohol use interact in determining the severity of violence. This has been done in Table 8.8.

Rates of injury in relatively close relationships were marginally higher when the assailants had been drinking, and there were more contacts with medical caregivers in the alcohol-related cases. A reversal of this slight tendency began with the middle category (those assailants who were known only a little or hardly at all), especially with the remedial contacts, but on the whole the results are inconclusive. The main finding in the comparison between the first two groups of familiarity is that there were higher levels of injury and curative action when the assailants were less well known to

TABLE 8.7. Injuries and Medical Activity in the Most Recent Episode of Physical Violence, as Related to Gender of Victims of Male Assailants and Drinking by These Assailants

	Victim was injured	Victim contacted hospital, doctor, nurse	Victim took or applied medication
Total ($n = 450$)	26%	11%	11%
Male assailant ($n = 377$)	28%	12%	12%
Female victim ($n = 143$)	21%	8%	6%
Assailant not drinking ($n = 67$)	18%	2%	6%
Assailant drinking ($n = 68$)	21%	12%	3%
Male victim ($n = 232$)	33%	15%	15%
Assailant not drinking ($n = 85$)	33%	14%	17%
Assailant drinking ($n = 124$)	31%	15%	14%

the victims, regardless of alcohol use. The indiscrimination hypothesis does not receive the slightest bit of support from this comparison.

When we get to the events in which the victims did not know the assailants at all, we can see that the patterns were totally and strongly reversed: 26% of violent incidents with drinking assailants led to injuries, compared to 73% when the assailants had not been drinking ($\chi^2 = 18.12$, $df = 1$, $p < .001$). As might be expected, rates of medical consultation (27% vs. 12%) and medication (31% vs. 7%) followed the same pattern. Whatever the explanations for this pattern, the indiscrimination hypothesis now receives some support in a roundabout way from the fact that there was a clear hierarchy of seriousness of violence (measured in all three ways—injury, care seeking, and medication) from close relationships to remote ones when the assailants had not used alcohol, but that this pattern did not hold true in events where the assailants had been drinking.

Comparing only the two extreme groups in Table 8.8 (the assailants known at least fairly well and the total strangers), we can see that both sober and drinking assailants caused more injuries and more injury-related medical activity when the adversaries were total strangers. However, the differences were much greater when the assailants were sober: 73% compared to 11% for injury ($\chi^2 = 20.59$, $df = 1$, $p < .001$), 27% compared to 1% for seeking of medical care, and 31% versus 6% for the use of medication. These findings are, of course, strongly in line with an indiscrimination effect of alcohol. On the other hand, typical alcohol-related and sober contexts (and related probabilities of intervention, etc.) may still play a role in these patterns, but this possibility cannot be satisfactorily tested with the present data.

TABLE 8.8. Injuries and Medical Activity in the Most Recent Episode of Physical Violence, as Related to How Well the Assailant Was Known to the Victim and to Drinking by the Assailant

	Victim was injured	Victim contacted hospital, doctor, nurse	Victim used some medication
Total ($n = 450$)	26%	11%	11%
Assailant not a relative or family member ($n = 299$)	27%	11%	11%
Assailant not drinking ($n = 134$)	30%	11%	13%
Assailant drinking ($n = 165$)	25%	11%	9%
Assailant known very well or fairly well[a] ($n = 132$)	13%	5%	5%
Assailant not drinking ($n = 74$)	11%	1%	6%
Assailant drinking ($n = 58$)	16%	9%	5%
Assailant known a little or hardly at all ($n = 64$)	39%	17%	19%
Assailant not drinking ($n = 34$)	38%	21%	15%
Assailant drinking ($n = 30$)	40%	13%	23%
Assailant not known at all ($n = 103$)	39%	16%	13%
Assailant not drinking ($n = 26$)	73%	27%	31%
Assailant drinking ($n = 77$)	26%	12%	7%

[a]Does not include the victim's relatives or family members.

Perhaps it can be concluded that there are some tendencies toward alcohol-related indiscrimination with regard to the closeness of the relationship between antagonists who are not related to each other or members of the same family. On the other hand, interactional rules of physical aggression applied to the gender of the victim by a totally sober assailant and one who has consumed alcohol prior to the aggression do not seem to differ. We will have to await the application of more powerful multivariate methods below for a somewhat more conclusive look at the patterns of influence.

In view of the societal interest in marital violence and the seriousness of its consequences for the wife and the whole family (even across generations of offspring), this section of the chapter will be concluded by taking a brief look at the role of alcohol in determining the seriousness of marital violence. In order to "purify" the comparison, only the incidents in which assailants were completely sober and those in which the assailants had been drinking have been compared. In sober marital violence, 13% of victims were injured ($n = 46$), compared to 26% in violence where the assailants had been drinking ($n = 38$). In the former category, 4% of victimized spouses sought medical care and 9% took or applied medication, while the corresponding figures were 13% and 5% when the assailant/spouse had been drinking. None of these differences between the two types of incidents were statistically significant, but there was at least a weak tendency toward more serious violence when the assailant (in 93% of the cases, the husband) had been drinking. Larger-scale studies or studies focusing on the role of alcohol in marital violence are needed for more conclusive tests of the extent to which alcohol aggravates physical violence between spouses.

DETERMINANTS OF INJURIES DUE TO VIOLENCE

Rates of injury and medical activity did not differ greatly between situations in which alcohol was involved and situations in which it was not, even when the central and potentially confounding factors of the gender of participants and closeness of their relationship were controlled for. Consequently, no support has been found for a general severity hypothesis in these data.

A general indiscrimination hypothesis has not received much support, either. We have seen in Chapter 7 that the acts to which male and female victims were subjected did not differ in alcohol-related and non-alcohol-related episodes in a way that could be seen as supporting such a categorical hypothesis of alcohol effects. Now we have seen that the differences in gender-specific injury and medical care patterns were no smaller when the assailants had been drinking than when they had not. However, with regard to the other socially and interactionally important dimension, the closeness of the relationship between the adversaries, some support has been found for indiscrimination in the cross-tabulations studied above. This indicates that conditions may have to be specified for when alcohol-related indiscrimination occurs; that is, hypotheses regarding a relationship between alcohol use and indiscrimination may have to be made contingent on some additional factors, particularly the nature of the discriminatory cues themselves. The processes seem too complex to be easily projected onto a single dimension of discrimination–indiscrimination.

In this section of the chapter, logistic regression analyses are presented that have been designed to provide some more conclusive answers to the nature of the determinants of seriousness and discrimination in violent encounters. In particular, they have been designed to show how the determinant power of alcohol use measures up in relation to other factors. Table 8.9 shows the familiar attributes of the four most impor-

TABLE 8.9. Summary of Rank Order, Direction, and Statistical Significance of Risk Factors in Different Logistic Regression Models Determining Risk of Injury to the Victim in the Most Recent Episode of Physical Violence

Risk factor	Rank order/direction
Male victim	−3
Male assailant	+2
Victim aged under 30	
Assailant aged under 30	−4
Victim knew assailant very well[a]	−1*
Incident located in a private home	
Victim drinking	
Assailant drinking	

[a]Including relatives and family members.
*$p < .001$.

tant determinants of injury through violence: direction, rank, and statistical significance.

The closeness of the relationship between the victim and the assailant was at a level by itself: An assailant who was known very well to the victim was much less likely to cause physical injury in a violent conflict. By comparison, the other factors in the first four ranks had little influence, and they did not differ much from one another in strength. None of them reached statistical significance in any of the models tried. Drinking by assailant and by victim had extremely weak influences, and their beta coefficients hovered around 0 in the different models.

The findings of Table 8.10 clearly indicate that the types of acts committed had a very strong influence on the risk of injury. The miscellaneous acts included in the "other" category (including such serious acts as being shot, willfully run over by a car, etc.) had the strongest determinant power of the four potentially most serious acts included in the model. Punching, no doubt partly because it is predominantly aimed at the vulnerable and unprotected facial area, had the second strongest risk increasing determination, with the use of weapons or objects for hitting the victim following in rank. Kicking, since it is carried out with the lower extremities, is targeted more toward protected and somewhat less vulnerable areas of the body (unless the victim is lying down).

Alcohol use by victim and assailant clearly neither increased nor decreased the risk of physical injury when considered in relation to relatively serious violent acts. The fact that the effects of serious types of acts have been controlled for here adds some assurance that any relationship between assailant's alcohol use and injury would not depend on the

TABLE 8.10. Alcohol Use and Different Acts of Violence as Determinants of Physical Injury in Most Recent Episode of Physical Violence, According to Logistic Regression Model

	β	p
Hitting with weapon or object	+0.76	.0170
Punching	+1.07	.0001
Kicking	+0.65	.0285
Other violent acts[a]	+1.70	.0004
Assailant drinking	+0.02	.9526
Victim drinking	−0.15	.6463
Intercept	−1.98	.0001
Likelihood ratio test of goodness of fit	$\chi^2 = 40.18$, $df = 33$, $p = .1820$	

[a]Does not include the relatively mild acts of slapping, throwing of objects, and grabbing, pushing, or shoving.

choice of violent acts by a sober as compared to a drinking assailant. (Moreover, I have already noted in Chapter 7 that drinking by the assailant did not have much effect on the choice of acts in any case.)

Thus far, the only exception to the lack of support for the *severity* hypothesis as measured by risk of injury is to be found in the events with victims who had consumed very high amounts of alcohol (see Table 8.6). Among these victims, the risk of injury was highly elevated at a statistically significant level (despite small subsamples). Very high consumption could to some extent be an indicator of victims' membership (and possibly that of assailants as well) in subgroups or subcultures with excessive alcohol use and a higher prevalence of relatively extreme violence. No good discriminating data on alcohol consumption by assailants could be obtained in this study, but assessed "drunkenness" did not cause any excess of injuries or medical consequences.

DISCRIMINATION ON THE BASIS OF GENDER AND CLOSENESS OF RELATIONSHIP AS REFLECTED IN INJURY RATES

According to the logistic regression models (which both satisfactorily fit the data) on which the risk estimates of Table 8.11 are based, there was a fourfold increase in the risk of physical injury for a male victim (aged 30 or over) when encountering a well-known male adversary who had been drinking, compared to one who had not. Among women of the same age group in violent conflicts with a male of this description, the relative risk was about twofold. On the other hand, there was a *decrease* in the risk of injury with a drinking assailant in more distant relationships (as has already been determined in the cross-tabular analyses), and this decrease was stronger among women than among men. The highest risk of injury was found among women who were assaulted by sober male strangers (0.61) and the lowest for victims attacked by sober well-known assailants (0.08 among male and 0.11 among female victims).

From the risk estimates of Table 8.11, standardized estimates of tendencies were calculated for (1) gender discrimination and (2) relationship (or familiarity) discrimination, when the other factor (relationship and gender, respectively) has been controlled for—a useful exercise, since, for example, women tend to be victimized more often in close relationships. This allows a more direct examination (compared to the summary of findings shown in Table 8.9) of the discrimination patterns related to injury for these two central factors, since situations in which the assailants were drinking have been compared to those in which they were not.

The risk estimates of injury caused by male assailants (when their victims were over 30, although this did not make much difference), standardized by the familiarity of an assailant, were as follows for these men and women:

	Assailant sober	Assailant drinking
Male victim	0.30	0.37
Female victim	0.36	0.29

In this group of victims, men had a slightly higher risk of injury when their assailants had been drinking and women a higher risk when their assailants were sober. The differences were too small for generalizations, however. It is remarkable that even when the degree of acquaintance between the victim and the assailant was standardized, women in this group actually had a higher risk of being physically injured by sober assailants (29% as compared to 36%). For our purposes, the main point is that there was no tendency toward less discrimination on the basis of the gender of the victim in violence episodes prior to which an assailant had consumed alcohol.

When the gender distribution was standardized in a parallel fashion, the "purified" differences in injury rates caused by assailants who were very well known to their victims and those who were not (most of these were total strangers) were as follows:

TABLE 8.11. Male Assailants Only: Risks and Relative Risks of Injury as Related to Gender of the Victim and the Closeness of the Relationship between the Adversaries (Only Victims Aged 30 and Over), According to Logistic Regression Models

	Risk of injury to victim when:				Relative risk of injury to victim by drinking assailant over sober assailant	
	Assailant sober		Assailant drinking			
Closeness of relationship	Male victim	Female victim	Male victim	Female victim	Male victim	Female victim
Victim knew assailant very well	0.08	0.11	0.32	0.25	4.05	2.21
Victim did not know assailant very well	0.51	0.61	0.42	0.33	0.81	0.55
Likelihood ratio test of goodness of fit of the models used	$\chi^2 = 4.60$, $df = 4$, $p = .3307$		$\chi^2 = 2.66$, $df = 4$, $p = .6160$			

	Assailant sober	Assailant drinking
Assailant known very well	0.10	0.28
Assailant not known very well	0.56	0.38

Like earlier analyses, this analysis has led to the manifest conclusion that indiscrimination with regard to how well the assailant was known by the victim was linked to alcohol use by the assailant. Whereas close assailants would cause injury in about 10% of violent conflicts when sober, unfamiliar assailants (mostly total strangers) would do so in 56% of such situations. When the assailants had been drinking, the difference is much reduced (28% as compared to 38%).

As a by-product, this analysis has provided the estimated total injury rates for victims aged 30 and over, standardized both by gender of victim and assailant (since only male assailants were included) and by the closeness of their relationship. These rates were identical for situations with a drinking assailant and a sober assailant: 33%.

Let us now see what support has been provided by these data for the role of alcohol use in increasing the risk of more severe, and more indiscriminate violence.[1] Focusing on the violent behavior itself has indicated that the choice of acts does *not* point to *general* indiscrimination in connection with alcohol use: Violent acts chosen against male and female victims differed just as much when assailants were sober as when they had been drinking. It has also been found that discrimination based on the gender of victim, as measured by risk of injury, did not change with alcohol consumption. On the other hand, when judged by the risk of injury, the discriminatory power of familiarity seemed to break down when assailants had been drinking. Therefore, for both gender of victim and degree of familiarity, the analyses in this chapter have essentially replicated the findings from the analyses of the choice of violent acts. Experimental tests of these conditional forms of indiscrimination seem called for.

There is no general support for the severity hypothesis in the present analyses. The standardized injury rate estimates were identical for drinking and sober assailants, and the highest rate was actually found in sober conflicts when the assailants were strangers or near-strangers. Since the

1. It has not been possible to test hypotheses regarding alcohol's role in *instigating* open aggression or violent reactions after alcohol use with the current sample of episodes. A closer look at episodes of severe anger and episodes of alcohol use will permit approximate tests of such elicitation hypotheses in the second monograph referred to earlier.

measures of indiscrimination used here (type of act and injury) coincided with the criteria used for severity, there are indications of the same type of conditional relationships as with indiscrimination.

It should be stressed that the present results have been based on episodes of violence that were not weighted by the probability of individuals' being involved in, or settings' being the scenes of, aggression or violence. Samples of violence that occur in specific subcultures with more extreme drinking habits, such as "skid row" social milieus, could possibly yield a distinct relationship between violent acts or injury and the use of alcohol. The amounts of alcohol consumed by members of such subgroups would also be considerably higher than those in the present general population sample, and processes specifically linked to high BAC levels might enter the determination of acts and injuries. This would explain the differing patterns found in some studies of violent crimes (Roslund & Larson, 1979; Wolfgang, 1958; Tardif, 1967), although an exacerbation of violence after drinking is not a pervasive finding in studies of violent crime and extreme users of alcohol. On the other hand, to the extent that there are sober encounters in alcoholic subgroups, they may be as likely as drunken encounters to result in aggression, violence, and injury. In order to test such a specification of this particular link between alcohol and aggression, we need special studies on these populations. Parallel analyses to the ones conducted here could also be carried out on violent crime data if sufficient and systematic information were collected via interviews and other methods. Such interviews may yield some more distinctly alcohol-related patterns with regard to both indiscrimination and severity, since they would largely involve a different type of population of episodes and actors, and the amounts of alcohol consumed would generally be higher.

9

Alcohol in Human Violence: Findings and Explanatory Frameworks

In this final chapter, I summarize the main findings from the analyses of the role of alcohol in episodes of violence from one Canadian community. A broad framework for constructing a theory that explains a heightened risk of aggression in connection with drinking is presented. It is argued that such a theory needs to be coextensive in important respects with a general theory of behavior under the influence of alcohol. As preparatory groundwork for the theoretical discussion, I also discuss additional conceptual and methodological issues related to the study of episodes of violence and, in particular, officially categorized violent crime. This discussion includes a criticism of the narrow theoretical scope in the traditional study of naturally occurring violence and its connection with alcohol use.

SUMMARY OF FINDINGS

Alcohol use was pervasive in the violence experienced by the residents of the study community. Over half of the most recent occasions on which they had been subjected to physical violence were preceded by alcohol use on the part of the assailants and/or the victims themselves. Moreover, in 42% of the violent crimes that occurred in the city, either the assailant or the victim or both adversaries had been drinking (and the 42% figure is without question an underestimate of the true level of the presence of alcohol). The separate proportions of victims and assailants who had been drinking in these events were as follows: (1) in the violent crime study, 31% of assailants and 26% of victims; and (2) in the interview study, 51% of assailants and 30% of victims.

We now have some evidence that, at least in a cultural sphere where alcohol is implicated in criminal violence, it is also abundantly present in day-to-day violent confrontations. The relationship between alcohol use and severe aggression, as reflected in studies of police and court records and in emergency room samples of injured persons, does not seem to be mainly an artifact created by biasing selection processes. Related to this, we also have evidence from this study that the statistical link is not limited to any specific, relatively small group or subculture of society that is overrepresented in official records of violence, even though such groups probably lopsidedly imprint their drinking and other behavior patterns on findings from any true incidence samples of aggression episodes.

The present data also indicate the existence of demographically categorizable groups with risks of alcohol-involved aggressive encounters above those derivable merely from their drinking frequency—for example, young adults, and in particular young men. Their heightened risk of experiencing aggression in different forms persisted in a number of settings. The information available in this material is not sufficient to identify the types of factors that explain this concentration among demographic segments of the population, but there are numerous potential candidates. Several are related to the substance of alcohol: typical amounts consumed at a sitting, drinking speed, length of drinking occasion (which allows or demands social interaction at potential high-risk positions on the blood alcohol curve), and so on. In all likelihood, we are here dealing with a determinative interaction between at least alcohol's more direct and unalterable pharmacological effects, and the semiotic and generally cultural status of alcohol use and drunkenness in these groups.

Still another finding of this study is that drinking by assailants had no statistically discernible effect on any of the violent acts chosen by them in episodes of violence. Neither did the alcohol use of assailants have any effect on risk of injury to the victims. The rate of injury to the victims was not related to any type of alcohol involvement (except for a statistically unsatisfactory cross-tabular indication of a heightened risk when the victims had consumed relatively large amounts of alcohol). It follows from this that no increase was found in the *severity* of violent acts when the assailants had been drinking. There were indications in the data of less *discrimination* in the use of violent acts after alcohol use. It was also reflected in injuries inflicted on the victims. However, this tendency was restricted to discrimination with regard to how well an adversary was known by a victim. With regard to the gender of the victim, discriminating use of violence by a drinking assailant was at least as pronounced as that by a sober one (such as it was). This finding contains rather clear evidence of the continued importance of conditional social-contextual cues and normative factors in the determination of types of aggression and physical violence after drinking.

As a general conclusion, it can be said that once aggression occurs in connection with drinking, it has the same general character of a "guided doing" as in sober conflict. Nonspecific "indiscrimination" and "excessiveness" *may* be more characteristic of determination in the initial stage of conflict, in the processes involving instigating cues and cognitive issues in angry arousal, and in the processes by which these instigations produce open conflict. Once the conflict has led to open violence, indiscrimination is not *generally* evident, but seems to depend on the discriminatory criteria. In other words, obliviousness, inattention, or "loss of inhibition" with regard to discriminating characteristics may be more pronounced for certain victim and setting characteristics than for others. (In addition to stable victim and setting attributes, discrimination-relevant attributes of the victim include signs of and behavior related to pain and injury in the adversary.) For this to be the case, *cognitive* factors (in a broad sense), and the effects of alcohol on cognitive functions, must be central in the explanation of the characteristics of violence linked to alcohol use.

There may still be special subpopulations in which wanton indiscrimination is found after the use of alcohol. There may also be levels of consumption at which indiscrimination or arbitrariness in the selection of forms of overt aggression is seen, and the choice of physically violent acts, normally grounded in the perception of the discrimination-relevant attributes of the victim, changes. However, it seems that such high consumption levels are so rare and/or relevant subpopulations so small in the type of general population studied here that they do not affect the characteristics of alcohol-related violence in the total population.

The present study seems to have found what MacAndrew and Edgerton (1969) call a "within-limits clause" in drunken comportment. Moreover, in drunken violence this clause seems to be invoked under some fairly common conditions of the same type and magnitude as in sober violence. In the most general terms, what I have found in studying violent acts (and, somewhat more inferentially, in analyzing injury rates) is the intrinsic dependence of behavioral "alcohol effects" on the social context and on the behavior and characteristics of the other interactants in the situation. Violence is a form of guided behavior, with rules and expectations that are applied and generally followed despite at times very intense arousal states. This has been expressed by Prus (1978) after reviewing a number of studies of deviant behavior: "Taken together these studies suggest that human violence has both a self-reflective and an interactive quality" (p. 53). It has been found in the present study that this quality of guidedness does not change abruptly but persists even when an aggressor has been drinking. Some changes in the application of such rules seem to occur, but this is probably a gradual process and depends on the nature of the rules. The exclusively "internal" determination postulated by explanations invoking "disinhibition" or "catalysis" does not validly describe the processes at work.

The direct implications of these findings for research and theoretical strategies are fairly general but central. From the findings on the prevalence of alcohol use in connection with violence in the general population of the community, we can conclude that the connection between alcohol and aggression is present in large segments of the general population. This means that we should not just be on the lookout for special physiological, psychological, and social processes linked to subgroups of the population, such as "skid row" alcoholics and violence-prone individuals. Psychological experimentation has (often seemingly by default) used a comparatively inclusive research strategy by choosing non-deviant subjects and corresponding theoretical universes, whereas social research has been more "problem-oriented" and more attentive to extreme phenomena and correlated groups of actors who exhibit deviant patterns of alcohol use or excessive violence. Both approaches are, of course, valid. What we need is a greater balance within each of these empirical traditions, as well as their general integration into a joint approach.

Another implication for both theory and empirical study that is evident from the present findings on the characteristics of alcohol-related violence—and one that should come as no great surprise, were it not for the force of prejudicial paradigms—is that in the study of alcohol use and especially the study of behavior "under the influence of" alcohol, we are in fact not only studying alcohol. Several types of empirical contingencies, many in themselves extrinsic to the use of alcohol and its effects, determine central behavior tendencies in connection with the use of alcohol. Many of these contingencies determine behavior after drinking in largely the same way as they determine behavior in a sober state. It further follows that alcohol's effects on perception and cognition mediate differences between drunken and sober conduct, since such contingencies typically must be appercepted by the drinker in order to wield their influence. No doubt some of these effects are based on the semiotic status of the social phenomena linked to alcohol use. This further underscores the importance of cognitive changes occasioned by the use of the substance.

The next section describes the strong thematic forces that intervene when explanations of alcohol-related violence are sought in empirical study and theory construction.

THEMATIC ONE-SIDEDNESS: OVEREMPHASIS ON AGGRESSION

Let us now enter into a discussion of considerable theoretical interest. Links of alcohol to discrimination–indiscrimination with regard to affectively *positive* acts were not examined in the present study. Neither were possible changes in the intensity of such acts after drinking (as a parallel to the study of the severity of violent acts). Such data would probably provide important theoretical clues. There is qualitative evidence in the present survey data that positive affect displayed toward the "wrong" person in a drinking situation, such as when a wife dances too intimately with a man other than her husband, can lead to friction and aggression in some cases. (This is part of the elicitation of alcohol-related aggression via interactional processes, which, judging from qualitative data in the present study, seems to be a central pathway connecting drinking and aggression.) In fact, this is what experience has taught many of us: Indiscriminate displays of positive affect increase after drinking. It prompted Ogden Nash to his well-known empirical generalization: "Candy is dandy, but liquor is quicker."

Unsystematic evidence accumulated from festive social contexts indicates that a great deal of rather indiscriminate affectionate behavior of various types occurs after drinking. Office parties, victory celebrations, stag parties, and other gatherings include disproportionate amounts of such behavior, ranging from innocent hugging and kissing to licentious conduct. Indeed, an important function of many such occasions is that they provide settings (and handy excuses) for such indiscriminate behavior. The following excerpt from one of the present study's observational sessions in a community tavern provides an illustration of positive indiscrimination. It also illustrates typical issues in alcohol-related conflict, because the show of affection is viewed as inappropriate—or, to put it more analytically, is displayed by the wrong kind of person in the presence of the wrong kind of persons in the wrong kind of social context (thus it yields several criteria for discrimination that are not satisfactorily met).

> The sequence of events took place between 12:20 and 1 A.M. in a tavern that was relatively high in aggressive encounters. Harry, who was in his early 20s, was seated with his parents. Lucy, a woman in her early 30s who was sitting at another table, walked over to Harry and hugged him. He introduced his mother, and Lucy shook her hand; when he introduced his father, she gave him a hug and a kiss. She then gave Harry a kiss and stayed at the table, talking to him in a very warm conversation. Turning her attention to Harry's mother, she started hugging and kissing her and Harry's father, saying, "I love you." She then walked back to her table, while Harry's parents looked at each other in disbelief and started talking about Lucy.

> Harry joined in, explaining how he met her and so on. In the meantime, Lucy moved to another table and grabbed a male in his 60s by his arm, gave him a hug and a kiss, and put her arm on his shoulder. Another man at that table was trying to get her attention and said something to her. Lucy replied, pulled his beard, and went back to her table. There she put a glass of beer to somebody's mouth, necked with another patron, and danced around with still another one. After a short absence, Harry's parents returned. His mother seemed upset and very concerned, sitting with a Kleenex in her hand.

This type of data is on a level with everyday observations, and Lucy's behavior cannot strictly be attributed to effects of alcohol. We need to know, in a systematic fashion parallel to the present analyses of violent acts, whether the types of affectionate acts that are discriminatively used in sober contexts (depending on the other person's gender, the extent to which the other person is known, the relative social status of the other person, the presence of other people, etc.) are also discriminatively used after the consumption of alcohol. For theoretical purposes, we also need to know whether some criteria of positive discrimination are affected more by alcohol use than others are.

This brief deliberation on the role of alcohol in displays of positive affect brings us to a discussion of the constriction of theoretical scope that is part and parcel of (1) the thematic force of violence and aggression and (2) the concentration of "real-life" research on occasions of aggression (the dependent variable) with no balancing study of episodes of alcohol use (the independent variable) and affective behavior in these episodes. Even in experimental research, where the episodes studied are intrinsically defined along the manipulated independent variable, there is an unfortunate tendency to concentrate exclusively on the measurement of behavior indicative of negative affect, while more positive interactional behavior in the same situation is neglected. This, I argue, occurs at the expense of theoretical extension and integration.

The stark label of "violence" or "violent crime" provides a vigorous thematic structure for our cognitions of phenomena, and thereby conceals elements of behavior that allow other types of categorizations of the interactional sequences preceding or concurrent with aggressive acts. In this way, the label often hides important aspects of human guidedness that are also present in the episode, and blocks important potential avenues for theoretical development. The strong thematic structure is further strengthened by the convenient sampling units and sampling frames used in the study of real-life aggression; these are almost exclusively made up of episodes of physical violence. This is very evident in extant studies of the relationship of interpersonal aggression to alcohol use. The exclusive use of samples of violence episodes in such studies limits the conclusions drawn and theoretical interpretations made. They provide a deficient base for many central analyses. This is so for two main reasons.

First, the selection of the samples is by definition carried out along the presumed dependent variable; that is, these are samples of *occasions when (aggression or) violence occurred.* This fact imposes restrictions on the assessment of the explanatory and predictive value of potential independent variables. Along the dependent variable, only *concordance* figures—such as percentages of violent crimes that were preceded by alcohol consumption on the part of the offender and/or victim (the standard measure of total alcohol involvement)—can be calculated. Even under the best of circumstances, we are in essence left with the logic of "case-control" methodology, which has been justly criticized as an epidemiological research method. The concordance between the two variables under the condition of different values of the third, such as the alcohol involvement of assailants in different age and gender groups, can of course give us preliminary clues as to multivariate causal connections. I have made some use of this possibility in the present research. However, even this type of analysis is relatively rare in the studies based on reports of violent crime, and it is impossible in the overwhelming majority of victimization studies because they do not ask about alcohol use (to the extent that they ask questions at all about specific incidents of violence). In addition, characteristics or consequences of violence can be studied using violence episodes as sampling units in the way that determinants of violent acts and injury have been studied here, but expanding the range of episodes for study would greatly enhance analytical possibilities.

If we are interested in estimating the risk-increasing (or, more ambitiously, the causal) role of alcohol and the role of other potential risk-increasing or risk-reducing factors as they relate to the *instigation* of aggression and violence (and this is perhaps the most central question in the study of alcohol-related aggression), we would do well to select samples along the presumed *independent variable* of alcohol use and not (exclusively) the dependent variable of violence. The proportion of alcohol involvement in different types of violent events, even if accessed from complementary sources or using different methods, will not, for instance, tell us whether certain characteristics of alcohol use situations or alcohol users are overrepresented in incidents of violence. Thus no assessment can be made of the potential risk-increasing or causal significance of these factors in eliciting aggression and violence. Central questions on the role of alcohol in the elicitation of frustration, anger, overt aggression, and physical violence cannot be asked. A sampling of alcohol use episodes would also provide us with a parallel to the experimental studies on aggression, which essentially create controlled drinking episodes and add manipulable characteristics that are designed to elicit a sufficient level of aggressive responding.[1]

Second, in addition to making use of drinking occasions for sampling and analysis, a more general *sequential* view is needed of the process whereby violence develops from conflict incitement or frustration through arousal and overt aggression to the use of physical force, and finally ends in some form of resolution of the violence episode. This sequential view should influence sampling considerations (again in open opposition to the thematic dominance of physical violence), since it will enable a look at the role of alcohol in different stages in the development of conflict. In this way, more isomorphic models of the determinative processes of alcohol-related aggression and physical violence can be constructed, and questions can be answered as to the role of alcohol in the elicitation of frustration and conflict, in the choice of overt aggression as opposed to other behavior or coping alternatives, in the escalation to physical violence, and so on. (This can be accomplished in addition to the study of alcohol's role in determining indiscrimination in the choice of targets or acts of violence, and in determining the severity of the violent behavior—the two functions that have been examined here.) I shall not enter into a detailed discussion of this aspect of broadening the sampling base in the study of alcohol-related aggression here. Instead, I hope to return to it in another context.

Samples taken of the first stage in this sequence (i.e., drinking episodes) provide much-needed corrective data. Contrary to the common scientific focus on aggressive behavior displayed in connection with drinking, such material shows that other types of affective behavior typically predominate in alcohol use situations. (This probably holds true even for many drinking occasions that include aggression.) Here basic description and/or a naive naturalistic orientation devoid of paradigmatic prejudices will rectify some empirical and theoretical misconceptions. Table 9.1 shows different types of mainly affective behavior displayed by at least someone in a respondent's company at his/her most recent drinking occasion in a home and in a public drinking place (as observed and reported by the Thunder Bay respondents of the present study).

Clearly, behavior usually linked to positive affect predominated. However, the results presented in Table 9.1 are not representative of the

1. A major problem in using this approach exclusively is that a great many drinking occasions will have to be sampled in order to obtain a large enough sample of situations in which aggression of the required severity took place. A combination of samples of drinking events and aggression events in the same study is probably the best strategy available at this time for assessing the role of alcohol use variables and other factors in the determination of naturally occurring aggression.

TABLE 9.1. Behaviors Displayed by at Least One Person in the Respondent's Company at the Last Drinking Occasion in a Private Home and in a Public Drinking Place

Behavior	In a private home ($n = 741$)	In a public drinking place ($n = 693$)
Laughing	70.8%	78.2%
Hugging or backslapping	9.7%	8.3%
Kissing, fondling	9.7%	6.9%
Showing off, bragging	4.2%	6.8%
Arguing, quarreling	4.9%	3.7%
Crying	3.4%	2.7%

Note. Only occasions at which at least one other person was drinking with the respondent are included.

behavior one would find when visiting the taverns and bars of the community (or when randomly intruding into private homes). The reason for this is that infrequent drinkers and their infrequent drinking patterns have been overrepresented in the results: The drinking events of respondents who drank once a month and their (perhaps equally temperate) drinking friends have been given the same weight as those of daily drinkers and their (on the average much less temperate) drinking companions. In another type of sampling procedure, designed to directly mirror the behavior encountered in drinking groups in public drinking places, the results given in Table 9.2 were obtained by pairs of trained observers during 600 hours of systematic observations in 28 local taverns and bars in the study community. The observers, working in pairs, recorded running accounts of behavior at randomly selected tables into a tape recorder. The results shown in this table, however, were based on structured coding sheets with ready-made categories of behavior, which were filled out immediately after each 3-hour observational session.

In Table 9.2, tavern and bar patrons have been represented in the proportion to which they spent their time in these settings. This means that, for example young community residents and especially young men have been overrepresented in proportion to their numbers in the general population; so, probably, have problem drinkers. Anyway, this table shows the comportment one would find when randomly visiting the public drinking places of the community at random times during their hours of business and roughly weighted by the numbers of patrons present at different hours. Here, as in the respondent-based results shown in Table 9.1, positive affect dominated. Even the aggression exhibited was mainly of the playful kind. This type of empirical balance in the study of

TABLE 9.2. Behaviors Displayed by at Least One Person in Randomly Sampled Drinking Groups (Two or More Persons), as Recorded by Observers in the Public Drinking Places of the Canadian Study Community

Behavior	(n = 645)
Laughing	78.2%
Shaking hands	22.3%
Backslapping	16.1%
Hugging	9.5%
Kissing on cheek	8.5%
Caressing (not erotic)	6.5%
Kissing on mouth	6.4%
Necking (erotic)	2.2%
Playful aggressive behavior	15.5%
Bragging, showing off	12.7%
Arguing, quarreling	10.4%
Pushing, shoving	4.0%
Other physically aggressive behavior	3.1%
Threatening gestures	3.6%
Crying	1.4%

behavior facilitates theoretical extensions in the study of alcohol's relationships with aggressive behavior.

Some behaviors in drinking contexts could thus be described as affectionate, others as good-humored or kind. Still others could carry labels such as generous, impulsive, or simply "emotional." Although they are probably more frequent than aggression, these types of alcohol-related behaviors reach us through the mass media much less often than is the case with aggressive encounters. In order to do so, they must be outrageously odd or funny, or must be seen as contradicting prevailing stereotypes regarding typical or expected behavior by certain categories of people. At least the latter is true of this description of the behavior of British nannies in Toronto restaurants:

> British nannies out on weekend tears have raised so much hell that the Bayfront Restaurant, near the Royal York Hotel, imposed a ban on them.
>
> They sing and yell and talk dirty. They have emptied ketchup bottles on the tables. They have filled waitresses' pockets with chopped onions. They have fled without paying. . . . (Jim Foster, *Toronto Star*, March 15, 1983)

Although these types of behavior can create a nuisance, they seem harmless enough. However, they are as much "caused" by drinking as the serious phenomena that are vastly better represented in our scientific focus. The possibility that they are subsumable, in some causally relevant ways, under the same theoretical categories as serious aggression found in connection with the use of alcohol should receive our analytical attention. Whether a drinking event with the same starting points evolves into aggression or harmless revelry, or both, will undoubtedly in part depend on situationally variable factors (including the behavior of other individuals in response to revelry—again a case for the consideration of social interaction and breaches of normative rules in the instigation of alcohol-related aggression). Idiosyncratic or random situational factors often seem to determine the seriousness of the outcome, and, on the basis of this, the dominant social categorization of an individual episode.

Aggression and violence are strong thematic conceptualizations in the structuring and interpretation of human behavior, and this in part explains the common selection of sampling universes. The thematic force is evident from the pervasiveness of aggressive themes in fiction and their prevalence in accounts from real life, such as those in the news media. Even in descriptions of aggression episodes, including drinking-related aggression, this thematic hegemony disguises thematically disparate phenomena in drunken individuals' apparent motivations, fluctuations in their affective behavior, and the behavior's multiple characteristics (recklessness, disregard, obliviousness, whimsicality, etc.). These types of behavioral factors may contain more valid explanatory potential than is inherent in the simple designation of an event as an instance of violence, and the consequent selection of information to fit this highly consequential theme.

It has been noted for sober circumstances that increases in aggression and hostility are not necessarily accompanied by decreases in behavior indicating positive affect (Nowlis, 1965). This has been borne out for alcohol use conditions in experimental research. Murdoch and Pihl (1985) found in an experiment that both positive and negative interactions were more common after drinking than in sober conditions. In a study of dyadic social interaction, the drinking subjects of Smith, Parker, and Noble (1975) showed increases in the affects of elation, giddiness, and happiness over the placebo condition. In addition, there were some indications of an increase in hostility, and a highly significant increase in total emotional expression. On the side of positive emotion, Pliner and Cappell (1974) found that subjects' mood was positively affected by alcohol in social situations, and subjects who received alcohol in an experiment conducted by McCollam, Burish, Maisto, and Sobell (1980) reported higher levels of positive affect over non-alcohol-consuming subjects. These examples showing high levels of positive affect after drinking could be multiplied (e.g., Connors & Maisto, 1979; Ekman,

Frankenhaeuser, Goldberg, Hagdahl, & Myrsten, 1964; Hartocollis, 1962; Jones, 1973; Myrsten, 1971; Vuchinich, Tucker, & Sobell, 1979).

Freed (1978), Russell and Mehrabian (1975) and Baum-Baicker (1985) have reviewed studies on the effect of drinking on mood and emotions. A few studies have found no emotional effects at all, and others only negative effects; there are clear indications that blood alcohol concentrations (BACs) are highly relevant in this determination, as is the position on the ascending or descending BAC limb. I shall not discuss the possible theoretical implications of these findings further, but only note that positive affect and fluctuations between positive and negative affect have been found to increase after alcohol use compared to sober conditions in experimental settings, where many confounding factors that trouble studies of natural episodes (as in the findings of Tables 9.1 and 9.2) have been controlled for.

In scientific reasoning on the subject, alcohol-related violence has been assigned to a different domain of discourse from general drunken comportment.[2] As a consequence of this scientific partitioning, theoretical extensions have not been drawn between aggression and other types of behavior that are more common in drinking situations (at least in general populations) than is aggression; it has seemed that aggression is aggression and should be studied as such. This one-sidedness in framing may be related to the seriousness and consequentiality of the scientific attitude (and its funding sources), which have hindered the explanations of drunken comportment from freely ranging between displays of both positive and negative affect and related conduct. It may also be related to the strict moral boundaries between the social problems related to alcohol use and the rather harmless mirth that is more typically connected with drinking. Moral circumscriptions may have impeded theoretical inclusiveness. This is not a unique phenomenon in the field; Kilty (1982) has argued that the uncritical acceptance of certain presumed effects of alcohol on human behavior are ultimately "rooted in moral prescriptions." As the manufacture, distribution, and consumption of alcohol and their consequences are matters of political and financial concern, there is the additional danger that research on the substance will bow to ideological and economical considerations (Heath, 1988a, 1988b; see also the rejoinder by Room, 1988).

2. This does not seem true in everyday conceptions of these phenomena. In the eye of the general public, drunken aggression is typically viewed in the same matrix of possibilities of action as, for instance, affectively positive behavior. There is abundant anthropological evidence of the wide range of behaviors observed and expected in connection with drinking; Taylor (1979), for instance, reports that the Aztecs called pulque "four hundred rabbits" in an effort to relay the variety of behaviors linked to its use.

THEMATIC SCREENING: OVERSIMPLIFICATION OF DRUNKEN BEHAVIOR

It is argued here that the research material available from episodes of aggression is too closely screened according to the dominant theme of aggression or violence (by the researchers or by independent documenters) to allow a sufficiently wide theoretical scope. As a countermeasure, what could be called "sequential disaggregation" of such episodes is called for. In such a strategy, sequences of events that lead up to the commission of physical violence would be documented as "themelessly" as possible. This description would include the whole range of affective behaviors displayed in the episodes and the action sequences leading up to these. This research activity not only ought to be carried out on the "objective" behavioral level, but should also encompass the symbolic, semiotic, and transactional dimensions of drunken interaction (and also sober persons' interaction with intoxicated persons). As part of such an effort, a microsociological framing in the analysis of intoxicated behavior would probably be useful.

Violent crimes committed under the influence of alcohol, although they characteristically include interaction sequences that can be labeled "aggressive" by any definition of the term, are too often replete with evidence of affectively idiosyncratic ideation and whimsical behavior to deserve that straightforward, one-dimensional label exclusively. From a theoretical point of view, the typical thematic screening leaves out not just "white noise," but also important clues as to the links between drinking and aggression.

In our thematic labeling and in descriptions of sequences of acts or events, we generally take the most consequential or culturally salient element of the sequences and build up a meaningful theme (or "scenario"). This helps us to cognize, understand, and study the episode, actor, and behavior. This process occurs much in the same way as it does with written fiction and staged interactions, as brilliantly expounded by Erving Goffman in his many important contributions to the understanding of human behavior (e.g., Goffman, 1959, 1961, 1963, 1967, 1971, 1974). (Were there not significant parallels with real life, we would not be able to understand and appreciate fictional representations.) Having done this thematic cognizing of staged representations, we judge how convincing they are by assessing how well the acts, interactions, and characters display the projected theme or themes. In real life, however, the characterizations that are available to us via contexts and themes are more variegated and not as easily determinable from the more inclusive context (e.g., from what happened before and what happens afterwards). In real-life interactions there are no titles or headlines, and no written interpretations or commentaries of the author's intent are available. In fictionalized human action and interaction, thematic and contextual cues are deliberately planted within the context presented to the audience. If biographies of the main characters are made available, they are explicitly or implicitly (but almost always deliberately) built up to suit and support the chosen themes. After all, the themes and characters are more often than not designed to be understood and appreciated. Even ambiguity of behavior, context, and thematic content is usually created for a purpose.

By contrast, thematic structurings of ongoing situations and interpretations of ongoing behavior in real life are very complicated processes, and typically several potential competing themes are applicable in any single instance. As participants or observers of an interaction sequence, we choose one or another thematic possibility on the basis of culturally and personally salient cues. Many such interpretations will never be, and can never be, verified as correct or mistaken. The understanding of *past* real-world behavior and interaction often benefits from post hoc thematic screening, and such activities preoccupy us intermittently in daily life. (This may all be linked to the economy needed in memory processing.) For scientific purposes this type of screening can be quite misleading, though, since it almost inevitably disregards the effects of nonthematic (or "microthematic") situational factors. Often the most salient theme-constructing cues are provided by the end result or resolution of an episode. Sometimes this is aggression, a powerful thematic cue; in reports of violent crime, it is the self-evident main theme. Such reports (both as written by the police and as provided in the news media) are thematically edited, and much material of potential explanatory importance has been deleted. After all, the (institutionalized thematic) reason for the police to write a report on human encounters including violence is that violence occurred.

I illustrate this screening process with a sequence of activity that is exclusively classified as violence; the description of the sequence (from a news report) contains conduct auxiliary to this theme. However, other, at least supplementary, thematic labelings are possible. Even in the thematically edited version presented here, it is possible to discern other types of affective behavior, which, however, cannot (and from a moral point of view ought not to) compete with the thematic force of serious aggression. The newspaper account deals with the trial of a man who, after drinking heavily for several days, raped a woman in her 20s. Before the rape occurred, he had made threats to his common-law wife, from whom he had separated a few months earlier. On the day of the rape episode, he paid a visit to her place of business, but she had left the building because of his threats:

> Allan, armed with a shotgun, went away and drank a bottle of whisky before he returned to the building and entered a rear door which leads to an apartment occupied by the rape victim and her husband, a couple he knew casually.
>
> The husband answered the knock on the door and was confronted by Allan, who said if he didn't let him in he would "blow his head off."
>
> Allan then drank a beer while he talked of his problems.
>
> Allan tied up the husband in the bedroom and took the wife to the front room, where he began to fondle her and warned her he would kill her husband if she didn't co-operate.
>
> Allan placed the shotgun on the floor, pointed at the victim, and forced her to commit sexual acts before he raped her.
>
> When he was finished, he asked her to put his arms around her and said, "That's all I wanted, was for someone to put their arms around me."
>
> Allan then apologized to both the husband and wife for what he had done, but a few minutes later struck the husband on the side of the head with the shotgun.
>
> The husband was knocked unconscious and Allan told the wife he was dead.
>
> Meanwhile, the woman began struggling with Allan and finally managed to grab the shotgun with both hands.
>
> Allan then told her she could leave.
>
> The woman ran from the apartment and flagged down a passing motorist.
>
> Police quickly surrounded the building but Allan didn't surrender for several hours. (*Toronto Star*, January 26, 1979)

Categorizations in scientific endeavors should not stem from cultural salience, but from a need for a more general theoretical focus. In an area dealing with socially problematic or deviant behavior, this needs to be specially emphasized. From the point of view of variable formation and hypothesis testing (not to speak of legal processing), it is necessary to use simple one-dimensional labeling of social episodes. It is perhaps too easy to take over institutionalized labelings in studying morally, legally, and administratively categorized phenomena such as violent crime. In scientific strategy, it is necessary to stop at crucial points or systematic intervals and try to cast an unbiased eye on the phenomena themselves, naturalistically. This may provide us with causally relevant observations that are not easily subsumable under, for example, the simple descriptive labels of aggression, violence, or deviance, or under postulated processes such as disinhibition, but that in the end may simplify explanation by subsuming a greater variety of drunken behavior under one theoretical umbrella.

In the sequence of acts by the rapist in the news story above, we can discern an affective indeterminateness or affective fluctuations possibly connected to the use of alcohol. From a theoretical point of view, this may be a preferable and primary thematic structuring of the episode. This indeterminate or fluctuating nature of behavior is also illustrated by a patron observed in one of the taverns of the study community.

Four patrons were sitting at a table in a tavern known to be high in aggressive displays. The attention of the observer was focused on Jordan, a male native Indian in his early 40s, who seemed moderately intoxicated.

At 11:15 P.M., the table was visited by Orwell, a male Caucasian in his late 50s on his way out from the tavern. He held Jordan's hand, and they spoke with their faces close together. It seemed that Orwell was giving Jordan a kiss on the cheek before he left.

11:20 P.M.: Jordan pulled Jane, a native Indian woman in her mid-40s and one of the four patrons at that table, toward him. He first grabbed her arm and held it, and then put his arm around her shoulder, pulled her toward him, and said something to her. He released her after a minute. She seemed a bit reluctant to be held this way, but not too reluctant.

11:50 P.M.: Jordan left the table and went to sit at another table at the back of the room. He beckoned to Jane to join him, but she remained seated at the old table with two men.

11:59 P.M.: Jordan was sitting at still another table at the bar and showing off to Jane by picking up his table with one hand.

12:06 A.M.: Jordan and Jane were talking across the room to each other. Jordan's words were not friendly. He made some ambiguous gestures, rather like salutes, to Jane. Jane was waving to Jordan to return, while Jordan was pretending he had a rifle in his hand and was pointing it all over the room.

12:15 A.M.: Jane was repeatedly waving to Jordan to return. His only response was to tell Jane to shut up.

12:31 A.M.: Jordan was walking around the room, stopping at various tables and asking for a cigarette. At the last table that he visited, he was pushed away very violently by the person he asked, and he almost fell to the floor.

12:36 A.M.: Jordan returned to sit with Jane.

12:39 A.M.: Together, Jordan and Jane fished around in a grocery bag that Jane had brought with her. They fished out a big hunk of ham and went around asking the other patrons to buy it for $3.00. No one wanted to, but eventually a waitress bought it.

12:46 A.M.: Jordan had left his table and was wandering around again. He walked to the doorway that separated the ladies' and escorts' section from the men's section. There he encountered Blackhat, a native Indian aged about 30, who had previously been sitting at his and Jane's table and remained seated there after Jordan left. Jordan now grabbed Blackhat by the arm and pulled it back. Blackhat responded by punching Jordan in the face. Jordan then punched Blackhat in the face. Jordan wiped his nose and checked his hands for blood; he was not bleeding. He returned to the table.

12:51 A.M.: Jordan had some harsh words with Jane. He stood up and hit Jane quite hard in the face.

12:55 A.M.: Jane was holding Jordan's arm. It was hard to tell whether this was a sign of affection or whether Jane was holding the arm as a defensive gesture so that Jordan could not slap her again.

12:58 A.M.: Jordan and Jane were holding arms and hands affectionately; they were relaxed. Then the situation appeared to change. Jordan got rougher and began pushing her back and forth. It was obvious that what was once affectionate was not so any more.

1:00 A.M.: End of observational session.

Witnesses to the above situation would most likely label this sequence thematically as aggressive behavior interspersed with sequences of behavior indicating positive affect. (However, in a background–foreground switch, it could also be seen and labeled as affectionate behavior interspersed with aggressive sequences.) If the violence were considered serious enough to be recorded by the police in an occurrence report, the expressions of positive affect would without doubt in most cases be edited out altogether, and so would much of the relatively neutral behavior. Also, in the common reader's and the common researcher's mind, the social consequentiality and thus the thematic salience of this sequence of events are firmly lodged in the displays of aggression, and this would determine the most likely labeling of this strip of activity. In explaining alcohol-related behavior, however, the most fruitful theoretical structuring of the sequence would perhaps be "affective fluctuations" or "heightened affectivity." This may begin to lead us toward valid explanations of a great deal of the aggression that occurs under the influence of alcohol, as well as drunken comportment generally.

All the variegated affective and behavioral themes evinced in connection with alcohol use (and suggested by such descriptive terms as aggressive, serious, wanton, silly, risky, inconsiderate, selfish, obnoxious, harmless, celebratory, affectionate, etc.) should lay equal claim to our theoretical attention. Also, in studying and explaining an increased risk of violence in connection with drinking, we should seriously consider the fact that if we were to seek correlations between alcohol use and events of extreme happiness, goodwill, revelry, and so on, we could well find these to be as high as the correlations between alcohol use and aggressive encounters. There may even be a fairly high representation of both types of affective behavior in the same interactional sequences. In addition, we may find a reasonable clustering of different types of affective behavior among certain types of individuals or groups of people, and more pronounced fluctuations in others. Such conceptualizations can lead to crucially relevant empirical research and may untie conceptual and theoretical "knots" in the explanation of drunken comportment.

TOWARD AN INTEGRATED THEORETICAL FRAMEWORK

Cognitive Guidedness versus Natural Determination

The discussion in the first chapter of this book has introduced two (in part contradictory) central structuring principles into the context of human intoxicated behavior: cognitive guidedness and natural, nonintentional determination. They are in their main features probably common to large segments of humanity. These cognitive principles compete in the explanation of human behavior. The inherent conflict between the two creates a dynamic of central importance to concept formation related to human activities. They clash with particular force in the perception of intoxicated behavior.

The two types of explanatory framings are intricately woven into the practical aspects of our lives and into its conceptual apparatus. The clash between framing principles is an ongoing one, and a great many of the concepts we apply to human behavior would not make sense if it did not exist. We continually test their applicability to the situations we encounter. In addition to providing the uneasy alternation that in some contexts is sufficient for a comical response, this conceptual tension is played out after the fact in resolving serious issues related to responsibility, intent, considerateness, sensitivity, and the like. Such concepts form a conceptual and (in part) epistemological web that derives part of its meaning from the two pre-empirical structuring principles. These frameworks are applied not only in innumerable private settings, but also in courts around the world, where natural determination is often invoked as an explanation (and excuse) for deviant acts and uncharacteristic behavior. It is similarly at the center of conflicts concerning the legal and medical status of the condition of alcoholism.

I have tried to illustrate how basically consequential and even tragic events linked to the use of alcohol can be seen as alternating between these two frames, with unexpected comic effects. Probably because alcohol is a chemical substance and an agent with predictable physiological outcomes, and even some foreseeable behavioral (e.g., psychomotor) consequences if ingested in large enough amounts, there has been a pull in the direction of the natural frame. This has been aided by the strength and power of research traditions in the natural sciences and general respect for their theoretical metaparadigms. However, intoxicated behavior in social contexts shows such great variation that in some observers' minds only the capriciousness of human free will has seemed able to explain it. There has therefore also been a pull in the other direction, that of guided behavior. This has led to an equally regrettable exclusive emphasis on cultural and situational variability of drunken comportment and to an interpretation of drunken behavior in a solely social-constructivist frame. Behind the situationally and socially variable façade, the relatively immutable effects of alcohol on, in particular, cognition have not been easy to detect.

It is the rather naturally/mechanistically causal that has had the upper hand in the explanation of drunken aggression. The mediating processes by which alcohol enters as a determinant of behavior have been put squarely in the domain of natural phenomena, with presumably predictable behaviors as outcomes even on the level of overt behavior (e.g., alcohol has been viewed as a "disinhibitor" or "catalyst" of aggression). Such formulations do not leave room for human guidedness and are totally immune to the influence of situational and interactional dynamics. A rather basic form of guidedness has been increasingly accepted in the explanations of the connection between drinking and aggression in the last decade and a half, but even this has been phrased too much in terms of the stimulus–response metaparadigm to allow true integration with attempts at thematic explanations of human conduct under the influence of alcohol.

Several researchers in the study of alcohol-related behavior have tried to correct scientific thinking in this regard, although disciplinary and paradigmatic boundaries have been hard to cross. Their influence has not reached the scientists who have worked under the guidance of natural-cause and stimulus–response paradigms. The most forceful corrective stance has probably been taken by MacAndrew and Edgerton (1969) in their extraordinary treatise on the cultural and historical variations in drunken comportment. In the light of the present study's findings, I must heartily concur with their position: "[W]hether addressing man's sober doings or his drunken doings, no theory of conduct that would gloss or ignore the role of discretion—and more generally, of meaning—in human affairs can hope to get very far" (MacAndrew and Edgerton, 1969, p. 89). However, their discussion of intoxicated behavior de-emphasizes the role of alcohol as a psychopharmacological determinant too much—in part, no doubt, because they attack a very general, vague, and rather simplistic view of intoxicated behavior.

Downplaying the basic effects of alcohol is widely characteristic of ethnographic studies in the area. This is in part understandable, since the focus of interest is on the institutionalized aspects of drinking and behavior in the context of drinking. However, important *distinctive* features of actual drunken comportment have often been lost in this way. Starting within the conceptual framework of the social sciences means that the points of reference have been exclusively taken from a sober viewpoint, with no room for the cognitive peculiarities of the drinker's phenomenal world and its behavioral and social-interactional outcomes. This is also a "reasonable" strategy in the study of social phenomena, since the standard explanatory arsenal—the socially institutionalized definitions and constructs—is to be found in the sober world (e.g., regulatory norms guiding and social functions served by specific patterns of behavior). Nevertheless, it is not a fertile strategy when used exclusively in the description and explanation of intoxicated behavior, and there is not much hope of arriving at isomorphic conceptualizations of the cognitive and phenomenal processes that determine drunken comportment in this way.

Such typically sociocultural-level theories are in effect totally indeterminate with regard to the most central questions that have arisen in regard to the connection between alcohol use and aggressive behavior in psychological research. I have already mentioned that the role of the physiological and psychological effects of alcohol is downplayed almost to the vanishing point. Even interactional processes—or, in general, possible risk-increasing conditional processes based on behavior cues typically available in the immediate situation (with threatening, provoking, and frustrating cues being of special importance)—or individual differences in reactions to alcohol are not addressed.

What MacAndrew and Edgerton (1969), Anderson (1978), Burns (1980), and many other social anthropologists teach us in numerous accounts of behavior in connection with drinking is that thematic guidance is very powerful (i.e., the perception and interpretation of thematic cues is fairly stable, despite variations in purely situational factors) in a majority of drinker–situation combinations. However, when a former leader of the Saskatchewan Conservative party celebrates his last day as official opposition leader by firing shots into the air from his .357 Magnum revolver and in consequence gets a $500 fine for possession of an unregistered restricted weapon and dangerous use of a weapon (*Toronto Star* [CP], November 17, 1979); when the commander of Bolivia's palace guard is arrested, removed from his command, and "placed at the disposal of a military tribunal for trial" for "a drunken attempt to enter President Lidia Gueiler Tejada's bedroom by banging down her door with a rifle butt" (*Toronto Star* [UPI], June 9, 1980); when a well-known American comedian dangles another movie actor out the window of an 18th-floor hotel window (Nancy Spiller, *Toronto Star*, December

12, 1982); or when a clergyman exposes himself to two young women on a train after having unsuccessfully tried to persuade them to strip for him (Sture Schött, *Aftonbladet*, Stockholm, Sweden, January 22, 1988), these seem like very individual acts of drunken folly counterproductive to any institutionalized and desirable stable definitions of status and self. (Most of these acts also seem to fall outside any definitions of permissible acts during "time out" in these societies.)

How would the "within-limits" functionality of drunken behavior, regardless of whatever social functions may be served, explain behavior that is clearly hazardous to the life and health of oneself and others? Perhaps the best illustrations of such behavior are found in anecdotes of drunks on airplanes who jeopardize the safety of all passengers. Drunken passengers who become so incensed because they are refused more alcohol that they harass cabin attendants in various ways are not uncommon. A relatively recent news report tells of a drunken man who started fairly innocuously with throwing soft clapbread at fellow passengers, and ended up threatening one of them with a raised bottle of vodka. He also tried to ignite his false teeth after pouring high-proof vodka over them, while the cabin attendant had to stand by with a fire extinguisher (Jan Lindström, *Expressen*, Sweden, May 19, 1988). Drunken passengers have also tried to force their way into the cockpit to talk to the captain and to have a stab at commanding the airplane.

We should, of course, not forget that really dangerous behavior among drinkers is rare. Harmless folly is much more prevalent. On the other hand, neither should we forget that such behavior is even rarer in a totally sober state. This is also reflected in the great proportion of accidents that are related to alcohol use in many countries (e.g., Cameron, 1977; Giesbrecht et al., 1989; Room, 1987; Smith et al., 1989; Wingard & Room, 1977). In addition to its psychomotor effects, which are relevant to most types of accidents, alcohol also increases the probability of risk-taking behavior (e.g., Cohen, 1960).

For our purposes, the most directly relevant phenomenon is naturally the serious violence that disproportionately occurs in connection with alcohol use. How does the "time-out" theory or any normative definition explain such phenomena? How does alcohol use as an excuse or as "deviance disavowal" get away from the obvious question of why alcohol is used in this way? Is everything based on social constructions without any grounding in observed behavior? Why is alcohol used in this way and not coffee, tea, or milk? Behind social definitions and thematic structures linked to alcohol, rather invariant natural-level effects of alcohol on human ideation, affect, and behavior are to be found, although the behavioral outcomes of such effects are situationally highly variable.

Meaningful social dimensions are relevant to the explanation of a great deal of alcohol-related aggression and physical violence. It is a solidly established fact that human behavior and interaction take place in a semiotic field with not only spoken or written words, but also objects, natural occurrences, human acts, human institutions, and so forth, serving as signs and symbols and providing meanings. There is no quarrel with this thematic determination of even intoxicated behavior. However, natural-level effects also enter these semiotic dimensions (e.g., Eco, 1979; Langer, 1951). Some of the meanings are established on the basis of observed natural regularities, as when rowdy, unpredictable, and aggressive behavior in connection with alcohol use assumes added semiotic potential, in that it can be used to hide sober and serious intentions. The use of alcohol as, for example, "deviance disavowal" does not preclude the reality of nonsemiotic causal (more concrete and resistant) relationships between alcohol use and aggression. In fact, the former in large part must rest on observed behavior regularities, or the possibilities for some symbolic and thematic connections between alcohol use and behavior would soon vanish.

A drinker not only learns the cultural meanings attached to alcohol and drinking; he also *learns about the basic effects of alcohol*, to a significant extent from personal experience (in addition to and interacting with what he learns from "what [his] society 'knows' about drunkenness"; MacAndrew & Edgerton, 1969, p. 88). Culturally, he may learn that he can use alcohol for, say, deviance disavowal if the prevailing beliefs and attitudes are such in his society, but this does not nearly exhaust the possibilities for planned utilization of alcohol effects. He also learns that by drinking, and by doing so in the right social context, he puts himself in a position where he will enable himself to do things he would not normally do. (I will argue in my upcoming monograph that one basic reason why people drink alcohol is that they seek to become more *situationally determined* than is possible when they are sober.)

Cultural themes evolve out of such realizations of situational effects, not just the other way around. Sitting in a dark corner of the bar with the girl he loves, a young man after a few drinks can more easily turn his romantic attentions toward her, excluding other distracting influences, and rather shamelessly pop a question or two. Thematic cultural strands, even some institutionalized ones, and combinations of such can probably be found in this setting (e.g., the music, the soft lights, and their combinations) and in this young man's behavior, but they in turn have partly evolved out of an awareness of the effects of alcohol. If we reach deep enough by removing layers of the semiotic superstructure of social meaningfulness, alcohol effects are sufficiently independent of any themes, cultural or other, to have many-pronged causal and semiotic significance.

This infrastructure is the reason why psychological experimentation on alcohol effects has external validity, although the situational and cultural range of present generalizations is still very much undetermined.

The social construction of reality emphasizes the structured, the routine, the expected—this is its function in human orientation to the physical and social world. When explaining such constructed social phenomena, we are by necessity moving within thematic structures. The ready-made terminology is not there for the unexpected, the idiosyncratic, the "theme-busting" behaviors. This is a weakness, especially when behavior tends more toward situational determination and thematic closure leaves a great unexplained residual variation. Nevertheless, the tendency to regard drunken comportment as based lopsidedly on natural-frame causation has been effectively counteracted by the thematic contributions from the social sciences, especially social anthropology.

It is not good research strategy to disregard, in explanations of individual behavior or data aggregated from distinct episodes of such behavior, what from a social thematic orientation may seem like random variations due to idiosyncratic factors. This is especially true when the main independent variable—in this case, alcohol in the bloodstream—is discretely distributed over individual organisms. A great deal of explanatory power is lost if individual and situational variations (including the blood alcohol levels of actors and other alcohol factors) are not taken into account for this purpose.[3]

Broad thematic explanations introduce thematic explanatory variables without attempting to examine even the mediating individual psychological and/or social-psychological processes through which the stated global factors determine individual behavior. Conversely, current psychological perspectives on alcohol-related behavior introduce factors exclusively on the individual level, without trying to vary socially variable factors in experimental manipulation or systematic sample selection.

3. There are, of course, strong justifications for the exclusive reliance on the thematic and global type of explanatory strategy when one is comparing homogeneous sociocultural units, such as small subcultures or small societies with *comparatively* little situational variation. Within such units, many situational factors—for instance, amounts consumed at one sitting, the type of company and activities, the functional importance of drinking (religious, festive, ritualistic, "bacchanalian," nutritional, etc.)—may be relatively stable. However, the sociocultural thematic structure by itself, without regard for the physiological reality of effects of alcohol within the organism, does not nearly suffice for explaining drunken comportment. This is especially true in larger and more heterogeneous groups of humans, where variations in alcohol variables, situational factors, and the definitions of drinking episodes are much greater. There, cultural themes do not suffice for defining the empirical variety of drinking episodes, as Simpura (1983) has found to be the case in his classificatory analysis of Finnish drinking episodes.

Contrary to general experimental research on aggression, where cross-cultural comparisons of, for instance, instigating factors or modeling processes have been carried out, differences between groups or societies have not received even peripheral attention in psychological research on intoxicated behavior. Hardly any cross-cultural replications or systematic comparisons between individuals from different demographic subgroups (e.g., gender and age) or subcultures have been carried out. The paradigmatic assumption has been that individuals from different cultures (and other socially definable units) and subjects in different social contexts are essentially interchangeable in their "reactions" to alcohol (at least under experimental conditions and manipulations), which of course implies exclusive natural-level determination.

Requirements for Integrated Models

The world is more complex, and also more integrated, than either of these metaparadigms (the individual distributive and the social thematic) would have it. The distributions, definitions, and interpretations of behavior cues are culturally and contextually determined, and thus we have to make use of culturally symbolic factors even in our distributive explanations of aggression and intoxicated behavior generally. Ideally, we should also attempt to do so in cross-cultural replications of experimental designs. At least, there should be an awareness of these complexities of meaning and social definition in interpreting experimental findings from different cultural spheres.

Natural-frame causality has its place in the explanation of drunken comportment, but not in the closed deterministic form that has tended to dominate explanations. Neither references to an unsubstantiated process of catalysis or disinhibition, nor simple stimulus–response schemata, fit even elementary observations of this behavior. Instead, models are needed that allow an integration of findings hitherto expressed in the divergent concepts of the two explanatory master frames: guidedness and natural determination. In order to lay claim to empirical validity, such models should at the very least isomorphically provide openings for contingent variations where such are observed in the empirical world. There is no paradox in the fact that natural-level occurrences in a living organism bring about changes that are of relevance to its orientational faculties, and there is no mystery in the realization that cognizing living organisms adjust to such changes and "make the most of the situation" as appercepted. Neither is there anything profoundly deep and disruptive of explanation in the fact that some natural-level occurrences and their psychological consequences are semiotically transformed, and in this way become meaningful and guidedly determinative on the cultural and interactional plane—that is, if we want to accept the world as it is. Naturalistic observation would probably reveal sequences of contingent determination and instances of human symbolism where the two master structurings meet unproblematically and rather imperceptibly in conjoint determination of concrete instances of drunken behavior and drunken aggression, but such empirically inspired integration has not been attempted. It is when we look at occurrences of alcohol-related behavior monolithically and nondynamically, and try to press them into one single type of paradigm, that philosophically tinged theoretical mysteries start rearing ugly aspects of their anatomy.

The thematic concerns of sociocultural theorizing in regard to drunken behavior have to be complemented by situational- and individual-level study and theory. As distant goals, integration of the two approaches and an openness to the possibilities of interactive causal processes between mainly situational and sociocultural factors will get us closer to valid explanations of alcohol-related behavior than will either strategy by itself. Drinking and drunken comportment are much more *integrally* woven into the social fabric than through mere normative or definitional thematic constructions, as expressed in concepts such as "time out" (MacAndrew & Edgerton, 1969) or "mythical drinking" (Falk & Sulkunen, 1981; Partanen, 1980), although semiotic constructs of this nature no doubt have determinant power (and in part spring from semiotic and cultural adjustments to natural-level effects of alcohol).

We cannot afford to keep the thematic and situational levels apart in explaining alcohol-related behavior, including alcohol-related aggression and violence, any more than we can do so in explaining sober conduct. Even less can we afford to perceive findings on one level as necessarily contradicting the other. Thematic structures themselves are in part present in the situational cues presented or otherwise available to the drinker. Sometimes thematic reminders are firmly imbued in the setting and the company of the drinker. At high enough BACs, even situationally supported thematic schemata may be lost, although there is evidence that they can be supported even at very high levels (e.g., Burns, 1980; Heath, 1958; MacAndrew & Edgerton, 1969; Washburne, 1961). Psychological theorizing and empirical work on effects of alcohol would do well to take greater account of contextual features of drinking situations, such as the broad and varying culturally meaningful themes in which they are embedded. Social theorizing and empirical efforts must on their part lose their fear of "reductionism" and take further account of situational and interactional factors. Surprisingly little work has been done on drunken comportment in the microsociological vein, as typified by especially symbolic interactionism and ethnomethodology. This approach would no doubt help us resolve some of the apparent contradictions between sociological and psychological findings and explanations of alcohol-related behavior.

The complexities in the determination of human behavior are well known. It does not get any easier to understand when we add the pharmacological influence of alcohol on the human mind, although natural-scientific paradigms and appealing pictorial representations (e.g., references to alcohol as a "catalyst," "trigger," "disinhibitor," etc.) have been invoked in attempted simplifications, as we have seen. If we pool the present knowledge available from different disciplines, there is convincing evidence of the crucial part played by alcohol's effects, by situational contingencies, and by social and sociocultural factors at several different junctures in accounting for alcohol-related aggression. At some point we have to stop regarding natural causation and human guidedness as independent (and sometimes rather arbitrarily alternating) explanatory structurings, as we seem to tend to do in explaining human behavior. Neither should they be seen as delimiting strictly parallel (and thus never intersecting) lines of empirical investigation. At this stage, the best strategy is probably to study, in both natural and contrived situations, *concrete* processes in which different types of determination intersect, overlap, or fuse.

As opposed to and as a possible background for the specialized study of deviant or pathological cases and extreme episodes of violence this book has looked at "normal violence" (although some extreme cases and reactions have been included due to the basically representative sampling of individuals and episodes). From the fact that the present study found no difference in the types of acts and in the prevalence of injury between violent victimizations in which assailants had been drinking and those in which they had not, we can draw the tentative conclusion that in the main, *transactional and instrumental functions underlie the definition and resolution of violent interaction even when aggressors have been drinking.* The objectives of violent behavior in the population studied were in large measure instrumental and transactional, both in a sober and in a drunken state. The present research also found that a conditional/contingent form of cognitive discrimination persisted in the violent behavior of drinking assailants. Therefore we can also state that resorting to physical violence and using specific acts, as well as the resulting pain and injury, do not in essential respects differ when assailants have been drinking and when they are sober. This probably holds true within a fairly wide range of consumption. With very high BAC values and in specific contexts, or with specific categories of individuals, this may not be a valid statement.

This brings us to the most basic requirement of a valid theory of intoxicated ideation, affect, and behavior, including drunken aggression. Such a theory must acknowledge the persistent orientational activity and the dynamics based on cognitive monitoring (within alcohol-induced parameters) that are typically exhibited in the behavior of a person who is under the influence of alcohol. The fact is simply that the drinker persistently tries to structure his immediate situation according to learned cognitive schemata and to make it meaningful, so that he can orient himself to it and to other humans present in the situation.

Generally, human beings structure their world according to what is important and salient to them in specific situations. Some of these structurings cover a very wide range of situations. The ones with the widest range could perhaps be called "existential" orientations: They deal with the meaning of life, religion, ideological convictions, and the like. Others are strictly situational. Among these are many simple instrumental ones; we only have to think of the small-scale structured instrumentalities involved in getting ready for work in the morning. Still other schemata have an intermediate status and apply (often by cultural definition) to a specific range of situations.

Human beings structure their world according to culturally and individually salient principles. They apply these structurings to situations and act on the basis of them. Cue values emerge from such structurings, but cues also determine orientational structures: There are constant interactions among and intermittent changes in cognitive structures. For example, the sight of an irate dog prompts orientations linked to self-preservation, and induces an instrumental search of means to escape the dog. In such a situation, a tree has a different cue value from that of a tree contemplated during a nature walk. Moreover, climbing the tree has no status relevance for most of us if we are alone with the dog, but it does in a situation where our neighbors are watching. Such orientational dynamics are also part of drinkers' phenomenal reality, and although predictable modifications probably occur, they are never totally subjected to the inanimate determination known from natural causality.

Let us also consider the following. In interacting with others, humans need to differentiate between categories of people in order to know how to perform their social roles, and in order to know what to expect in specific types of interactions with them. This holds true in school, at work, in family life, and even when drinking in taverns, although the specific structuring principles or schemata and their applications differ greatly between settings. The anthropologist Clifford Geertz (Geertz, 1973) suggests that such social-orientational capabilities are an intrinsic part of the human organism and that they have evolved over millions of years in the phylogenetic adaptation to a changing (and basically cultural) environment. Similar thoughts are increasingly expressed in the ethobiological study of human beings.

Numerous treatises have been written about structuring processes as they occur in a sober state—in the macrosociological area labeled "value orientations"; in microsociological analyses in part overlapping with "definitions of the situation"; and in minute behavioristic contexts squeezed into the concept of "goal-directedness" with little allowance for the cognitively variable. No systematic attempts seem to have been made to chart what types of ordering processes are characteristic of individuals who are affected by alcohol, or to study how these differ from such processes in a sober state. (This problem cannot be reduced to a question of alcohol-induced changes in affect or cognitive abilities.) However, we have seen that the need and the tendencies to structure and order one's world do not vanish with the first few drinks. Nor do the categorizing, structuring, and attributional principles that are applied in structuring situations seem to change very abruptly. In the interview data from the present study, we have seen this to be the case even with regard to the rather small-scale rules that regulate the nature of violent acts as they depend on the characteristics of the target of violence. Modifications take place nonetheless, and I have suggested that these modifications are in large part mediated by the effects of alcohol on cognition.

Theoretical conceptualizations in the distributive mode that explicitly suggest which actual empirical processes mediate between alcohol and aggression (e.g., that go much beyond perfunctory references to disinhibition of primitive or other inhibited impulses) have come forth, especially in the last decade or two (Cherek, Steinberg, & Manno, 1985; Hull, 1981; Pernanen, 1976; Steele & Southwick, 1985; Taylor & Leonard, 1983). In opposition to the "internal" disinhibition idea, these newer theoretical positions and the empirical studies issuing from them postulate cognitive guidedness through *situational* means in the production of alcohol-related aggression. Unfortunately, references to *thematic structures* in alcohol-related behavior are still predominantly couched in vague one-dimensional terms (inhibition, expectancy, etc.). Thus it is relatively common to find normative rules, practical contingencies, instrumental strategies, individual behavior patterns, presence of bystanders, psychodynamic processes, and other factors that decrease the risk of violence under some empirical contingencies all lumped summarily under "inhibiting factors" or "inhibition." In this way, social dynamics linked to aggression in connection with alcohol use are ignored. Through this projection into one dimensionality the role of alcohol in "disinhibiting" processes is basically mechanized.

Most social situations probably contain both inhibiting and facilitating (including truly disinhibiting) factors, and what should be accounted for at the most basic levels of explanation is how facilitating factors for the specific criterion behavior (in our case aggression) achieve predominance in some alcohol use situations. Moreover, both instrumental and symbolic uses of alcohol and its real, perceived, and socially defined effects also influence individual behavior and social interaction in connection with drinking. These cannot easily be subsumed under a stimulus–response paradigm, and certainly cannot be coded onto the inhibition–disinhibition dimension without a significant loss of meaning, explanatory power, and usefulness.

Both the relevance of interactional processes and the cognitive ramifications of alcohol use have been neglected in theories attempting to explain drunken conduct, although there has been a change for the better in recent years. Two very general and central facts should be taken into account in developing any theory of intoxicated behavior. First, if we accept the importance of human interaction and its cognitive determinants in the explanation of behavior under the influence of alcohol, *any* internal alcohol-induced process would only *in part* explain the occurrence of aggression in connection with alcohol use in the real world. Second, whatever the validity of the assumption that alcohol is a "mood modifier" through some relatively direct physiological effects on mood or affect, there should be no doubt that it is a "mind modifier" (and at least in this way exerts an influence on the drinker's emotional life). This is evident from scores of studies on the perception, attention, learning, memory, intellectual abilities, and other faculties of intoxicated humans.

Human behavior under the influence of alcohol is not exclusively determined by social definitions and social learning, and thus it is not subject to wanton geographical and historical variations. Nor are aggression and other behaviors solely determined by alcohol's pharmacological and physiological effects. Instead, the connections that we regularly find between alcohol use and the occurrence of aggressive behavior are the outcomes of several types of processes acting conjointly, dynamically, and even semiotically. Some component processes are direct natural-level outcomes of having alcohol in the biological system. Others are socially determined. Many of the latter have probably been derived through the semiotic activity (definition and interpretation) of generations of human beings who have based them on commonly experienced and observed effects of alcohol. Even the psychophysiological alcohol effects thus have a dual role. They are active directly, but they also appear in many symbolic disguises and are mediated through social definitions. Such semiotics are only in part covered by narrowly conceptualized expectancies of the drinker, which have recently received a disproportionate interest in experimental research.[4]

Human behavior is not exclusively determined either by great thematic definitions (historical, cultural, functional, personal, etc.) and rules (conscious or subconscious), *or* by situational, comparatively haphazard factors. It is determined by a mixture of both, and the study of the nature of that mixture should be very central to the understanding of all human behavior. In all likelihood, however, determination by situational factors is more prevalent under the influence of alcohol. Situationality, perhaps because it is rather easily subsumed under a stimulus–response paradigm, may in effect be one reason behind the pressure to regard intoxicated behavior as naturally determined. Increased situationality is partly why we decide to drink alcoholic beverages from time to time. Often these situational factors are such that they are conducive to atypical behavior including aggression and violence, but in some circumstances with stable situational stimuli (and clear-cut institutionalized meanings pertaining to the situational context), there may not be any detectable difference to sober performance (Pernanen, 1976).

In explaining the linkage between alcohol use and aggressive behavior, we are dealing with a mesh of pharmacological, physiological, cognitive, learning, social-definitional, social-interactional, and other factors. Some of these feed on each other, through natural-frame causality or through symbolic/semiotic processes. In addition, we should not make the mistake of assuming that the same types of factors are involved in explanations of all occurrences of alcohol-related violence. In some explanations the physiological processes connected with alcohol use predominate, such as possibly in rage reactions following alcohol use among persons with epileptiform temporal lobe abnormalities or in hypoglycemic states (e.g., Pernanen, 1976). In others, the social-definitional, cultural, and interactional factors are of prime relevance, and the present data have indicated that these may be very central in shaping the alcohol-related aggression that occurs in general populations.

Despite the obvious need to operationalize theoretical problems into a subject-based individual format for experimental testing, we must not lose sight of the basic fact that human aggression normally occurs in social and interactional contexts. Aggression is in most cases an interaction between two or more meaningfully oriented individuals trying to find and establish a congruent definition of the situation and to act in

4. There are other "pathways" in which the linkage between alcohol use and aggression is more cumbersome. Some of these are connected to the interactional disturbances caused by psychomotor, cognitive, and affective outcomes of alcohol use, and the transactional impact of these outcomes.

consequence of this definition. Related to this is the central fact that an aggressive incident, despite the thematic adjustments in, say, the condensed format of a police report on violent crime, is not a unitary phenomenon pervaded by aggressive feelings, aggressive intent, and aggressive acts by one or more participants. Alcohol makes its own characteristic mark on these processes, but very seldom do the participants totally lose their capability for guided behavior and their openness to situational contingencies. In a basic human manner, the drinker tries to gain needed cognitive control of the situation and to give it a meaningful definition in order to be able to act and react.

Instead of looking for generally applicable explanations of drunken demeanor grounded in very specific and unalterable effects of alcohol on the behavior level, we need explanations that take into account the wide situational and cultural variations observed in this conduct. We should also try to incorporate into our explanations empirical processes that are observable in the naturally unfolding world, and not be content with explanation of findings from controlled settings. By focusing in part on behavior in naturally evolving episodes, we will run less risk of neglecting important dynamic aspects of drunken behavior.

Even at this early stage of development in knowledge about the alcohol–violence link, we will have to accept that no *single* causal model will explain why alcohol is implicated in so much violence and other forms of aggression. Alcohol, drinking, and drunkenness are too much a part of the symbolic fabric of society to have remained on an innocent, uncontaminated, natural-scientific level, where only its pharmacological properties determine the behavioral outcomes of the ingestion of alcohol. Drinking persons perceive, think, act, and interact within the same definitional and interactional framework as everybody else. Their acts are contingent on cognitions and actions of others in their immediate situation and stable milieu, whether they are sober or intoxicated. A drinker's own cognitive functions will change with the ingestion of alcohol, but these functions will not cease until the final comatose stage, at which point the individual is not of much interest to the study of the determination of behavior by alcohol use anyway.

The ultimate observable end results—in the form of the covariation of per capita consumption of alcohol and rates of violent crime over time, and in the proportion of participants who have been drinking prior to episodes of violence—are composites of many different empirical processes. Some alcohol-induced processes actually decrease the likelihood of physical aggression, as when a high amount of alcohol incapacitates a would-be aggressor, or when alcohol in some circumstances leads to reconciliation between bitter rivals. These processes also have an impact on the total aggregated alcohol–violence relationship—in this case, by reducing it (Pernanen, 1981). To complicate things further, the set of processes comprising the reality reflected in total alcohol involvement percentages (see Chapter 2) is not by any means identical to the set determining the extent of covariation between per capita alcohol consumption and rates of violent crime.

In the combinations of, and the junctions between, natural-scientific causal determination and cognitively mediated links with symbolic processes and (social-)definitional givens, we shall probably find the most fascinating and theoretically fruitful of the variegated processes linking alcohol to aggression. In all probability, we will here also find links between drinking and other types of affective behavior besides aggression. In fact, there is not much hope of finding a relatively general theory explaining the relationships between alcohol use and aggression unless we find a valid theory of the influence of alcohol on behavior generally. In view of the fact that drinkers retain their basic inclination (and, indeed, their need) to orient themselves to their environment, this theory must include central premises derived from the effects of alcohol on human cognition.

We need to know much more about interactional and communicational rules and the transformations that these undergo (through *several types* of causally relevant processes) when at least one interactant has been drinking or is obviously intoxicated. We need theories that integrate the psychologically manifested effects of alcohol (especially on cognition) with the social–interactional fabric and the social definitions that structure our world—drunk or sober. In this way, we will also learn more about human sober behavior and its complicated web of interactional and communicational processes. Hopefully the findings and ideas brought forth here will serve to bring closer together the social and psychological study of aggression and violence, of which a considerable proportion occurs in connection with drinking.

APPENDIX A

Methodological Considerations: Representativeness of the Sample of City Residents, and the Validity of Responses

In this appendix, I first discuss the representativeness of the sample of Thunder Bay residents that was taken with the Henderson City Directory as a sampling frame in the way described in Chapter 3. The discussion includes (1) a direct comparison between the final sample obtained and census figures on some focal demographic characteristics, and (2) a look at attrition and its possible effects on some central findings concerning alcohol use and experiences of aggression. Second, I try to assess the possible impact of confidentiality aspects and related social desirability factors in the interview situation on the same clusters of data.

CHECKS OF REPRESENTATIVENESS

Census data are generally thought to reflect well the true demographic profile of any area, in part since the enumeration of individuals is based on a fresh geographical sampling frame of dwellings. The interview survey in the present study used listings of names and addresses of residents that had been obtained from such a frame. In addition a "mixed" area sampling was carried out of dwellings that had been listed as vacant by the Henderson City Directory. Substitutions were used if the selected respondents had moved from their addresses. Primarily because of the attrition rate of about 25%, it is important to compare this sample to the more complete census data available for the year 1981.

Demographic Representativeness of the Interview Sample

A comparison between the gender and age distribution of the interview sample of Thunder Bay residents, and that of the total community population as reflected in the 1981 Canadian census, is shown in Table A.1. It can be seen that the correspondence was relatively good except for an underrepresentation of the oldest residents in the interview sample. This resulted primarily from the decision to omit residents of nursing homes, old age homes, and other institutions from the sampling frame. For all intents and purposes, it can be said that the sample was representative of the community population aged between 20 and 69. An exploratory exclusion of the underrepresented population segment aged 70 and over did not alter the results for the total sample on any of several key distributions and estimates. Consequently, this subgroup has been included in all the analyses of the survey.

The distribution according to education of the community population aged 15 (not 20) and over and not in full-time attendance at a school was also available from census data. Residents with a relatively low educational attainment were somewhat underrepresented in the survey; there were 22.8% with less than a grade 9 education, compared to 29.1% according to the census of 1981 (Ministry of Supply and Services Canada, 1984a). At the other end of the educational scale, 30% of the respondents reported having at least some postsecondary education, compared to the census figure of 26.9%. Two factors probably explain most of this discrepancy. First, the census data pertain to the population aged 15 and over, whereas the present sampling frame excluded all residents under the age of 20. Second, as noted above, the oldest residents, who were also those with the least formal education, were underrepresented because residents of nursing homes and old-age homes were excluded. When these factors are taken into account, the distribution of the survey sample along formal education can probably be considered sufficiently similar to the census distribution (within the rough categorizations necessary to obtain comparability between survey and census data) to allow generalizations to the community population on this variable.

The representativeness of the survey sample has been further assessed via a comparison by occupational category. This comparison only included individuals who were gainfully employed at the time of the survey and the census, respectively. The overrepresentation of residents with higher education perhaps reflects the fact that occupations requiring a higher education were somewhat overrepresented in the survey. Three broad occupational categories (out of a total of 12) requiring higher than average education—(1) managerial or administrative positions; (2) natural and social sciences, law, and religion; and (3) teaching and related occupations—were represented to a proportion of 19.2% in the survey, compared to the census figure of 16.7%. On the other hand, five categories—(1) farming, fishing, forestry, and mining; (2) industrial production and machining; (3) construction; (4) mineral ore and metal processing; and (5) transport and

TABLE A.1. Distribution of Survey Respondents, and of the Total Community Population According to 1981 Canadian Census, by Gender and Age

	Male		Female		Total	
Age	Census (n = 41,595)	Sample (n = 489)	Census (n = 42,140)	Sample (n = 444)	Census (n = 83,735)	Sample (n = 979)[a]
20–24	14.5%	12.6%	14.1%	15.1%	14.3%	13.9%
25–34	24.9%	22.4%	23.6%	20.9%	24.2%	21.6%
35–44	16.6%	20.6%	15.8%	16.6%	16.2%	18.7%
45–54	15.8%	19.8%	14.8%	19.6%	15.3%	19.7%
55–64	14.2%	14.9%	15.1%	18.1%	14.6%	16.5%
65–69	5.3%	3.1%	5.9%	5.8%	5.6%	4.4%
70 and over	8.7%	6.5%	10.7%	3.9%	9.7%	5.2%

Note. Source for census data: Ministry of Supply and Services, Canada (1982). Percentages in some columns may not total 100% because of rounding.
[a]Weighted by gender. The unweighted number of cases is 933.

"other" categories (which include traditional blue-collar occupations)—were also overrepresented in the survey, the share being 41.4% as opposed to 37.1% in the census. The clerical, sales, and service occupations were the main ones underrepresented in the survey. (The census data for occupations have been taken from Ministry of Supply and Services Canada, 1984b.)

The divergences between the survey and census in regard to occupations were at least partly caused by random sampling fluctuations. Discrepancies in the matching of occupational classifications may also explain part of the difference. Some individual categories also presented special attrition problems. For example, people working in transport often had relatively irregular working hours, and thus were harder to pin down for an interview. In addition, the experience during the fieldwork was that some "bush" workers only came home on (some) weekends, and this created difficulties in arranging interviews; this would to some extent explain the underrepresentation in the category that included forestry workers. On the whole, however, these discrepancies appear to have had relatively little influence on important aspects of the survey. It can be stated in summary that the community sample, weighted for the initial lower sampling fraction of women and adjusted for their higher response rate, was sufficiently representative of the population between the ages of 20 and 69 on some central demographic variables.

Reasons for Attrition

Interviewers were instructed to make the first contact in person, but it was left to their discretion whether the next contact or contacts were made in person or by telephone. No actual interviews were conducted by telephone. The reasons for

TABLE A.2. Reasons for Attrition in the Community Sample

Reason	Number of attritions	Percentage of total attrition group ($n = 319$)	Percentage of total selected sample ($n = 1,252$)
Refused	235	73.7%	18.8%
Aged—unable	22	6.9%	1.8%
Sick—unable	17	5.3%	1.4%
Language difficulties	16	5.0%	1.3%
Away for the duration of the study	11	3.4%	0.9%
Incapable[a]	5	1.7%	0.3%
Never home/available	5	1.6%	0.4%
Other reason	8	2.5%	0.6%
Total	319	100.1%[b]	25.5%

[a]The category of "incapable" includes 3 persons (out of 5) who were too intoxicated to be interviewed.
[b]The total does not come to exactly 100% because of rounding.

final attrition are shown in Table A.2, percentaged with both the community sample and the attrition cases as a base.

Men were overrepresented in the attrition cases and among the final refusals. Female refusers were also somewhat more likely than male refusers to reconsider and assent to an interview later on in the fieldwork. The only attrition category in which women were clearly overrepresented were those who reported being too sick to take part in the study. The overall unweighted response rate for the survey was 74.5%; women had a somewhat higher response rate (78.1%) than men (73.4%). In the presentation of substantive findings of the survey, the responses of female respondents have been weighted up by a factor of 1.1 in order to make the sample correspond to the gender distribution in the community population aged 20 and over.[1] When the initial oversampling of males was taken into account, the corrected response rate for the survey was 75.3%.

ASSESSMENT OF THE AGGREGATE VALIDITY OF INFORMATION ON ALCOHOL USE AND EXPERIENCES OF AGGRESSION

Representativeness with regard to the first-stage sampling units does not necessarily imply representativeness in the second-stage units of episodes of alcohol use and aggression. No valid independent data exist for even the incidence and

1. In 1981, the proportions of men and women in the population of the community aged 20 and over were 49.67% and 50.33% respectively (Ministry of Supply and Services Canada, 1982).

prevalence of such episodes, let alone their specific characteristics. Thus I have used some more inferential measures of validity here. First, some data on the refusals and other attrition cases have been analyzed. This has permitted a rough assessment of the effect of biases due to attrition in the final survey sample on the information obtained regarding alcohol use and experiences of aggression. Second, some data from a mailed questionnaire sent out to most attrition cases after the completion of the fieldwork have been analyzed in a corresponding manner.

Reconsidered Refusals

Almost all the individuals who had been selected for an interview and who had refused to participate at first personal contact were later telephoned by one of five experienced interviewers, who tried to set up an interview. In this way 55 additional respondents were interviewed; they made up 19% of the original refusers ($n = 290$). Through this procedure, the response rate of the representative community survey (excluding the special Finnish sample) was increased by 4.7%. (These individuals are not included in the final attrition cases presented in Table A.2.)

Refusers who reconsidered showed a very low level of experiences of aggression, compared to the rest of the interviewed sample; in the preceding 12 months 6.8% reported having been subjected to violence, 1.7% to threats with a weapon, and 5.1% to verbal threats of violence. When these figures are compared to the second column of Table A.3, it is apparent that this segment of original refusers would not through their attrition have biased the results toward an underestimation of rates of aggression in the community.

Questionnaires Mailed to Attrition Cases

An attempt was made to get further data on the influence of attrition by mailing a brief questionnaire containing central survey questions to 255 of the 319 attrition cases, including 224 of the 235 final refusals and 38 of the other 84 attrition cases. Altogether, 77 questionnaires were returned; of these, 11 were unsatisfactorily completed or were obviously completed by someone other than the intended respondent. These were deleted from the comparative analyses. The remaining 66 completed questionnaires made up 26% of all questionnaires mailed out. Sixty-one of these were completed by persistent refusers in the interview survey. The return rates did not differ between men and women.

The mean number of reasons given for originally refusing the interview was considerably higher among the refusers who did not fill out the questionnaire (2.9) than among the ones who did so (1.8). This may be an indication that this segment of refusers was a largely untapped reservoir of the interview study, in that the interviewers did not persevere in the contacts with these respondents (which either would have resulted in interviews or would have led the prospective

TABLE A.3. Prevalences of Experiences of Aggression and the Proportion of Nonabstainers in the Interview Survey and among Respondents to the Questionnaire Mailed to Attrition Cases

	Mail sample ($n = 66$)	Interview sample ($n = 933$)
Victimized by violence in last 12 months	10.7%	9.4%
Threatened with weapon or object in last 12 months	3.9%	2.9%
Threatened verbally with violence in last 12 months	12.0%	6.8%
Drank alcohol at least once a year	91.5%	89.1%

respondents to give additional reasons for their lack of cooperation). Thus, the questionnaires were completed by individuals who were more likely to have become respondents in the interview survey than were the ones who did not respond to the mailed questionnaire. If this interpretation is correct, the individuals who mailed questionnaires constituted a biased sample of the attrition cases (mainly refusals), and generalizations to the rest of the attrition cases (or refusals) are perhaps not warranted. Nevertheless, they made up about one-quarter of the persons who refused, and thus they would have had a bearing on some of the potential bias due to this attrition factor.

The differences between the mail and interview respondents on some key variables were small, considering the limited sample size of the mail survey (Table A.3). Not even the difference between proportions of respondents who received verbal threats during the 12 months preceding the interview (12.0% vs. 6.8%) was statistically significant. The tendency toward a higher rate of drinking and experiences of aggression can to some extent be explained by the higher proportion of men in the mail sample (65% as compared to 52% in the unweighted interview sample). For present purposes, the central conclusion is that at least part of the nonresponse in the interviews did not seem to lead to major biases on key variables.

THE INTERVIEW SITUATION AND POSSIBLE SOURCES OF BIAS

Up to this point, I have discussed potential indications of biases arising from faulty sampling frames and attrition. Important biases may also have originated or been revealed only in the interview situation: recall errors and the social desirability effect (lying and shading of responses).[2] The possibility of recall

2. The distinction between these two sources of error is not as clear-cut as it may seem; related to difficulties of recall are greater possibilities of shading one's answers. The process need not be entirely on the conscious level.

errors will be discussed in a separate cross-cultural report on methodological matters, and I shall not enter into a discussion of this potential type of bias here. (There were no indications of major effects of recall on the nature of violence and threat episodes reported in the survey.) After a brief look at the length and time of interviewing and the interview situation, I examine some indications of the effects of (1) less than ideal confidentiality conditions in the interview situation, and (2) the interviewers' observations of hesitation in responding. These are linked to considerations of confidentiality and social desirability, and their relationship to responses to some sensitive questions and to the interviewers' judgments of undue influence during the interviews is discussed.

The mean duration of the interviews was 57.8 minutes, with a median of 55.0 minutes; it ranged from 10 minutes to more than 3 hours. Two-thirds of the interviews lasted between 40 and 70 minutes. Many of the questions did not apply to abstainers or to persons who reported that they had not experienced any violence or threats of violence since the age of 15, and with these respondents the interviewing time was naturally much shorter than with others.

Most of the interviews were carried out during the fall months of 1977. The distribution over the months is given in Table A.4. As for distribution over days of the week, surprisingly few interviews were carried out on weekends (8.6% on Saturdays and 3.9% on Sundays), and even Fridays showed a lower than average share of interviews (11.4%). By contrast, the interviewing was relatively evenly distributed over the other weekdays, with a mean of 19.0% of the interviews on these days. This probably reflects the weekly rhythm and preferences of our interviewers as much as respondents' wishes.

The months of interviewing contained several major holidays: Thanksgiving, Christmas, and New Year's. However, over 80% of the interviews had been carried out by the end of December, and any deviating patterns of alcohol use would not have affected the results appreciably. This was particularly true since the overwhelming majority of comparisons and other analyses were carried out

TABLE A.4 Distribution of Interviews over Different Months

Month	Percentage of unweighted sample ($n = 933$)[a]	Cumulative percentage ($n = 933$)
September 1977	15.3%	15.3%
October 1977	35.0%	50.3%
November 1977	27.9%	78.3%
December 1977	6.5%	84.8%
January 1978	7.2%	92.0%
February 1978	4.9%	96.9%
March 1978	3.1%	100.0%

[a]Percentages in this column do not total 100% because of rounding.

within the interview sample and not with outside statistical sources or other samples of individuals. The comparisons made with police record data referred to occurrences during a 12-month period, which means that ideally the date of interview would have had no importance. Recall may have had some effect on 12-month estimations of experiences of aggression, and seasonal fluctuations may thus have influenced results through the choice of interviewing date. Weekday of interview may also have had an effect on estimates related to amounts consumed and so forth, especially since such estimates were only requested in regard to the most recent drinking occasions. However, cross-tabular analyses of weekday of interview, time distance to most recent consumption, and weekday of most recent consumption did not reveal patterns of appreciable bias.

Projecting and Securing Confidentiality

Many aspects and consequences of alcohol use are viewed negatively or ambivalently in society. Some forms of drinking are actually stigmatizing, and people who indulge in these are met with disapproval, disparagement, or ridicule. Perhaps the clearest examples of these are alcohol use patterns that show addictive features and occur at the expense of familial or societal obligations. Also, drinking too much at one sitting and the inability to "hold one's liquor" are generally considered undesirable. Some other types of behavior found disproportionately in connection with alcohol, at least in the popular mind, are similarly disapproved. "Debauchery" used to be a common label for such activities. These considerations are all linked to the risk of obtaining invalid data through the rather obtrusive method of survey interviewing. The present study also faced the same type of difficulties (similarly reflected in "dark figures" in official recordings of violence) regarding the other major set of variables of interest: Aggression and violence also constitute a sensitive area of human conduct.

In order to prevent tendencies toward consciously biased reporting or refusal to respond to sensitive questions, a number of standard procedures have been worked out in survey research. Central in these efforts are attempts to convince the prospective respondent that his/her answers will be treated with utmost confidentiality and that the interviewer is a person to be trusted. In interacting with the respondent, the interviewer therefore must somehow display that he/she is not prejudiced against any of the behaviors under study, or at least understands that certain circumstances can lead to deviations from normative expectations. The interviewer may also have to convince the respondent that any qualms he/she may have are overridden by the importance of getting valid responses for the wider (in this case, scientific) purposes of the study.

At least three different concerns related to confidentiality are involved in the social interaction of the interview situation and potentially influence the validity of information provided by the respondent. The first pertains to the future handling of the information given by the respondent. To counteract apprehensions related to this type of confidentiality, efforts are made to convince the respondent that the data will be handled with utmost care once the interview has been completed. Usually, potential concern regarding this aspect of confidentiality is addressed with reassurances in an introductory letter to the respondent prior to the first personal contact by the interviewer. This was done in the present study. A letter was sent to each prospective respondent with assurances that all information gathered would be confidential; that only a very select few in the research team would have access to the information in an unprocessed and identifiable form; and that published results would only appear in aggregated form, with no individual responses reported in a way that would make it possible to trace them to individual respondents. These same reassurances were given orally by the interviewer at the beginning of the interview session. In addition, the completed interview schedule was enclosed in an envelope stamped "Confidential" and was sealed in the presence of the respondent. This envelope was shown to the respondent before the actual interviewing commenced. All interviewers signed forms binding them to strict confidentiality with respect to all information received during the interview. The only identification on the response form consisted of a five-digit identification number. The respondent was informed about these precautions before the start of the interview.

A second aspect of confidentiality with inherent threats to optimal validity is the presence of other people in the interview situation. Ideally, the interview should be carried out with no other people present in the same room or within hearing distance. Most often this can be accomplished, but sometimes the interviewer has to make compromises with the ideal in order to obtain an interview at all. This is unavoidable, for example, if the respondent does not know the language in which the interview is conducted and an interpreter is needed: this was the case in some of the interviews for the present study. With the data obtained in these situations and in others where third parties were present, some tentative assessments of the effects of the presence of other people in the interview situation have been made.

A third aspect of confidentiality with related social desirability potential is the interaction in the dyadic constellation of respondent and interviewer. Does the respondent feel secure enough to tell this stranger about things of which he/she may feel ashamed, or things that are so sensitive that he/she would prefer to keep them secret, even if they are completely alone and the respondent is confident that the information will not be leaked to anybody in any way? In the present study, flash cards containing fixed response alternatives to questions dealing with specific episodes of aggression and occasions of alcohol use were used. It was felt that reporting on domestic violence would meet with the greatest social desirability effects. Therefore, the relationship to the other person in the violent event, as well as his/her age and gender, the nature of the violent acts, and the like, were precoded on these flash cards (see Appendix B). In answering some of these questions, the respondent only read out letters or numbers referring to the alternative responses. In other questions (e.g., those asking about specific acts of physical violence), the interviewer read out an alphabetical or numerical code and the interviewee only responded with a "yes" or "no." The interviewer did not have the response alternatives written out in the schedule. No doubt some interviewers, after conducting a number of interviews, learned what responses some of these codes stood for; even then, however, the procedure probably served to reassure respondents about the confidentiality of their answers. This was the unanimous feeling of the interviewers in commenting on the use of the flash cards. It was also expressed in some of the written descriptions of the interview situation provided by the interviewers after each interview. This one is typical:

"Wife came, after interview had started, to listen and offer her opinion on one question, whereupon I pointed out that I had to have the respondent's opinions. She asked if it was all right if she listened, so I said it was suggested that respondents be alone, as someone else's presence might influence their answers. Anyway, she soon lost interest and left once we started talking in letters and numbers and she couldn't understand what the questions were about!"

The method of using flash cards for "blind" asking and coded responding applied to all three loci of confidentiality concerns discussed above, and most directly to possible social desirability effects in the interaction between respondent and interviewer.

Because there were no reliable aggregated data for checking at least the aggregate validity of the prevalence figures of violence and alcohol use obtained in the survey, more inferential methods had to be used to complement standard precautions and the use of confidential flash cards (none of which could be directly assessed in their effects on the validity of responses).

Possible Biases Due to Presence of Others in the Interview Situation

As part of the methodological assessment, the interviewers were asked to describe each interview and to provide a rating of some features in the interview situation with potential relevance for validity of responses after the completion of each interview. This was done on a separate one-page form (see Figure A.1).

Assessed Influence by Third Persons

In the training of the interviewers, it was emphasized that interviews should be conducted in private if at all possible. In order to provide an indication of the privacy in which the interviews were conducted, the interviewers recorded whether other people were present in the interview situation and rated the effect that they thought this had on responses. Another person was present at one time or another in 43% of the interviews, an unexpectedly high proportion. However,

Questionnaire No. ☐☐☐ - ☐☐

To be filled out by interviewer immediately after interview

1. Did respondent have any language difficulties? ☐
   1. A great deal
   2. Some
   3. None at all
2. Was somebody else present in the same room during interview? ☐
   1. All the time
   2. Some of the time
   3. Not at all → GO TO QUESTION 4
3. Did this seem to affect the answers given by respondent? ☐
   1. A great deal
   2. Somewhat
   3. Not at all

	Yes	No	
4. Did the respondent hesitate to answer some of the questions on alcohol use?	1	2	☐
On aggression or violence?	1	2	☐

5. Describe the interview briefly: ________________________________

____

____

____

____

FIGURE A.1. Form for postinterview assessment of possible biases.

in only 18% of the interviews was the other person present during the whole interview.[3] Another person was much more likely to be at hand when the respondent had at least some language difficulties. Somebody else was present in over 70% of interviews where there were such difficulties ($n = 72$), but in 40% of interviews with no language problems. In the former situations, someone else was present all through the interview in almost half the cases.

Unfortunately, the value of the information on the presence of other persons is reduced by the fact that it was not systematically ascertained who this third person (and possibly still others attending) was. The open-ended descriptions provided by the interviewers show that in many cases this third person was a small child whose influence on the interview consisted of interruptions, which distracted the respondent to some extent. On a few occasions, the interviewer even shared babysitting chores with the respondent during the interview. The following are some interviewers' notes on occasions with children present:

"The father [i.e., the respondent] had to frequently attend to two small boys, one of them a 'holy terror.' . . . A good interview in spite of difficulties of father with child interference."

"The respondent was very cooperative, even though she had trouble with her small child crying most of the time. She seemed concerned about alcohol abuse in the city."

"Teenage children sitting across the room watching TV, but not taking any notice of us and I'm sure couldn't hear us."

"Just interviewee's 6-year-old daughter who was home from school at this time. She was drawing and paying no attention to the questions."

"Small child ran out, and interview was interrupted by both of us going to [a local convenience store to fetch] the child."

The types of interview situations in which another adult was present only part of the time are exemplified in the following descriptions by interviewers:

"Husband came in to watch TV toward end, but didn't take any notice of us."

"Wife came in once or twice to get things as she was getting ready to go to work. They hadn't told me before, but near the end he said his wife had to be

3. In a relatively recent survey on alcohol use in Finland, 34% of interviews were carried out at least in part in the presence of someone else (Simpura, 1983). In an early alcohol use survey among residents of the Finnish countryside, Kuusi (1957) reported that someone else was present in 45% of the interviews, and was able to monitor the whole interview in 35% of all interviews. Usually, however, this type of information about survey procedures is not reported and analyzed even in relation to sensitive interview information.

driven to work, so I elected to stay and wait about 20 minutes at their offer instead of returning."

"Respondent was a charming, vivacious old lady—her mind alert and bright, well read, and up on the political scene and world events. Her daughter put in an appearance, but immediately left when she found things going so well."

"Daughter dropped in to leave her child to be babysat when I had almost finished the interview."

Sixteen cases of attrition were due to language difficulties. In most cases of difficulties with the English language, an interviewer could be found who spoke the respondent's native language. (In addition, the interview schedule was translated into French, Italian, and Finnish, and at least one of the interviewers was fluent in one of these languages.) In several interviews, a member of the respondent's family translated the questions—not a desirable procedure, considering the sensitive nature of some of the questions.[4] Below is a fairly representative selection of interviewers' comments from interviews carried out with one or more impromptu translators:

"The subject did not understand English well, so his daughter agreed to stay and translate. They appear to have a very good relationship, and she was very patient in explaining the questions and allowing him to think out his answers aloud. I was satisfied that the responses reflected his ideas and that he understood the questions."

"This was a difficult interview. Respondent could not speak English at all, although he could understand 'some.' His wife acted as interpreter, although her English was very poor. The interview was pleasant enough, but all questions had to be fully explained, and it took forever! Very nice people."

"Respondent had great difficulty with the language, and various child relatives and his wife helped with the interpretation. I do not feel that the presence influenced the answers at all, but I also feel that he had difficulty in expressing his feelings adequately and that some of his replies to the statement questions may not reflect his true opinions."

Most frequently, though, even when there were language difficulties, the respondent knew enough English to complete the interview without outside help. According to the assessment of the interviewers, 92.1% of the respondents had no

4. We may be victims of (sub)cultural bias in interpreting some information as sensitive for all subsegments of a society, especially a multicultural one. What is sensitive in some ethnic groups can very well be openly discussed within the family, and even with strangers, in others.

difficulties in answering the questions due to problems with understanding or speaking English (or Italian, Finnish, or French if the interviews were carried out in these languages); 6.2% had some difficulties; and 1.6% had a great deal of difficulty.

Even when there were no language difficulties, some respondents requested that someone else (most often a family member) be present. The interviewer had to accept this arrangement in order to secure an interview. In many of these cases, the respondents felt that their reading abilities, eyesight, or other capabilities (e.g., understanding of difficult words or recall of past events) would not suffice for the interview. In a few cases, the respondents just seemed to need the moral support of the presence of some other person.

> "The wife helped in reading. Interesting twist to interview. [The respondent was] pleasant and cooperative, slow-thinking."
>
> "Respondent suffers from Parkinson's disease, but insisted on doing the interview. He also could not read; therefore, his brother was helping by reading items on cards to him."
>
> "These two young ladies live together and work together as a team. Respondent said she had to be with her. Her companion just sat quietly by."
>
> "Respondent seemed tired, may have lost concentration near the end of the interview. Understood questions well. A very warm and friendly respondent. Wife helped with some dates; otherwise she did not affect respondent's answers."

In most cases the other person or persons did not take part in the interaction, even though present in the same room or within hearing distance in another room:

> "Respondent's wife was in and out all the time, but not in an interfering way, and it did not seem to influence the answers at all."
>
> "Respondent's girlfriend listened in, but she seemed to have been with him on most of the [aggression and drinking] occasions mentioned, and so she knew about them."
>
> "Respondent's wife was recovering from an accident and on the couch all the time. She did not interfere in any way. Respondent seems to live with gusto, hard-working and hard-playing."
>
> "Seemed very glad to participate. Husband was in the kitchen with radio on—interested in questions—no door to close. He only helped with question on income. Very affable."

The interviewers judged that the presence of a third person had at least some effect on the responses in about one-fifth of the interviews in which somebody else was present at least part of the time. This share was about 8% of all interviews. The influence appeared to be most prevalent in the interviews where the third person served as a translator of questions and responses. The interviewers estimated that 45% of interviews with language difficulties were such that the responses were somewhat affected by the presence of another person, whereas this was true for only 17% of the cases where another person was present but where there were no difficulties with language.

In less than 1% of the interviews in which another person was present did the interviewer feel that this influenced the responses "a great deal." This translates to 0.4% of all interviews. This low figure may in part be a reflection of a great proportion of children among those present. The share of interviews judged to be affected at least "a little" by the presence of an outsider was, as might be expected, at its highest when the presence lasted throughout the whole interview: 30% ($n = 160$), compared to 15% ($n = 230$) for those interviews where someone else was present only part of the time. The range in the assessed disturbance or influence on the respondent was great and varied in nature:

"The respondent was very young. Mother would occasionally come into the room or would listen at entrance. Difficult to say if this caused respondent to tone down some of his answers."

" Respondent's husband kept interjecting answers, but respondent seemed to keep to most of her original answers, with the exception of some disagreement over the number of persons present at the last drinking occasion at home."

"Mother listened and suggested with the TV on. Difficult with confusion of TV and mother, but daughter understood the required format and held her own."

"This young woman's father kept interfering and asking me unreasonable questions, to the point that his daughter was visibly annoyed with him. A very suspicious man."

When the respondent felt that pressure was exerted to change responses, there was sometimes a reaction:

"Interview went quite well, even though the respondent's wife was present and interrupted to answer for him. He took the initiative to tell her to 'mind her own business.'"

"Respondent told his wife: 'It's my interview. Go and see the kids in the bathtub.'"

Some unsystematic comments by the interviewers on the assessment sheets also indicate that the influence, especially when the third person acted as an interpreter, was most marked with regard to attitude statements and questions of judgment and opinion; it did not affect questions about factual occurrences, such as alcohol use and experiences of aggression, as much. This was what Kuusi (1957) found in some quantitative analyses in his by now classic study of drinking in the Finnish countryside: When another person was present, responses to questions on personal opinions were more in line with prevailing social morality regarding alcohol use, whereas there was no difference in information given on actual drinking behavior. In fact, as we have seen, the validity of factual questions was sometimes improved by the presence of a third person in the present study:

"I had called earlier with a previous appointment, but was left in the cold. This time the respondent was a little sheepish and had a tendency to minimize his drinking. His wife reminded him from time to time and kept him from deviating. A pleasant ordinary interview."

Unfortunately, information provided in the literature on surveys of alcohol use seems to have left the possibility of an increase in validity due to the assistance provided by another person at an impressionistic and anecdotal level. The experience from Finland, where (with the possible exception of Sweden) probably more alcohol use surveys have been carried out per capita than in any other country, indicates that this holds true also for this sociocultural sphere (T. Pöysä, personal communication, 1981). Kuusi (1957) noted that the spouse's presence aided in the recall and truthful reporting of amounts consumed, company at drinking occasions, dates, and the like. Moreover, joint interviews with two or more household members have been conducted in many consumer and victimization surveys in a deliberate attempt to improve validity of responses.

The most direct test of third-person influence, however, is through a comparison of the criterion behaviors, aggression and alcohol use. I institute such a comparison later, after looking at another type of assessment carried out by interviewers.

Assessed Hesitation in Responding to Questions on Aggression and Drinking

The interviewers were asked to make some additional assessments of occurrences in the interview situation. They were asked to record whether there was any "hesitation" on the part of the respondent in answering the questions on violence and drinking. According to the interviewers' judgment, there was at least some hesitation by 9.8% of the respondents on questions about personal experiences of violence, and by 5.6% on questions regarding personal use of alcohol.

Table A.5 relates the interviewers' perception of hesitation to the presence of other people in the interview situation. There was least hesitation by the respondents in the interviews that were carried out in complete privacy; about 10% of

TABLE A.5. Hesitation by the Respondent (as Assessed by the Interviewer) in Responding to Questions on Experiences of Violence and Personal Alcohol Use, According to the Presence of Other Persons in the Interview Situation

	Other person(s) present			
Hesitation in responding	At no time (*n* = 518)	Part of the time (*n* = 229)	All of the time (*n* = 162)	Total (*n* = 909)
No hesitation	89.6%	84.3%	85.8%	87.6%
Questions on violence only	5.4%	10.5%	6.2%	6.8%
Questions on alcohol use only	2.1%	2.2%	4.9%	2.6%
Questions on both alcohol use and violence	2.9%	3.1%	3.1%	3.0%

Note. Percentages in some columns may not total 100% because of rounding.

respondents in these situations were judged to have hesitated at least some time to either set of sensitive questions. When somebody else was present all through the interview, the proportion of respondents hesitating in their responses to these questions was about 14%. When someone else was present only part of the time, the proportion was minutely higher, about 15%.

These were hardly differences of any great impact on the findings; they were not even directly related to the duration of the presence of other people. Thus, this presence does not seem to have had any appreciable effect on the respondents' hesitation to answer potentially sensitive questions on alcohol use and experiences of violence. With the type of veiled questioning (involving flash cards and codes) on alcohol use and aggression employed in the present study, privacy may not be a decisive confidentiality issue. It is also possible that rapport between interviewer and respondent becomes somewhat less important when such a method is used, since the interviewer does not openly receive sensitive information. (However, the effects on readiness to respond that are related to the respondent's faith in the later discreet handling of the data still depend to a great extent on rapport with the respondent.)

Regarding the questions on alcohol use, there were some elaborations by the interviewers in the forms provided for this purpose. Often these included confidentiality concerns related to persons (or settings) other than the respondents themselves, as in this interview:

"The interviewee only hesitated to answer whereabouts of the bar where he had last encountered violence. Otherwise no hesitation. Very cooperative. Wife was present, but watched TV."

Instances of candidness regarding alcohol use were also recorded by the interviewer. In some cases these were prompted by the situation:

"Respondent said he is an alcoholic. He has been in an alcoholism ward several times—has quit for periods of time, but is on again. He drank three beers during the interview. I gathered that respondent drinks about 12 beers a day (morning, noon, and night) during the week and about 24 on weekend days. He was quite open and honest and willing to answer questions. He said his wife gets quite annoyed when he drinks so much. Respondent was beginning to stutter by the end of the interview—but wasn't at all aggressive. He said he didn't dare touch whisky because he couldn't handle it, so he drinks beer. He said he was quite 'wild' and got into lots of 'scraps' when he was younger, but has slowed down now—stays home and drinks."

"Respondent was intoxicated during the interview. He lives in a small crowded home with three children. His wife continually corrected him on the verbal response questions. . . . He and his wife were really concerned about the distance they have to travel to get a case of beer."

In a few instances, when respondents were judged to have hesitated to answer questions on violence, it was more often than not evident that they wanted to tell the interviewer the whole story, and explained or otherwise showed the cause for their hesitation:

"Respondent didn't want her daughter to hear some of the talk regarding threats in connection with question 26 [types of threats she had been subjected to since the age of 15]."

"[The respondent] was willing but unable to answer as fully as she wanted on violence, as her husband was nearby. She spent a lot of time thinking out her questions."

"The woman is remarried and had a violent first marriage, so she did not want her second husband to hear all her comments."

"A simple, noneventful interview with veiled mother–son violence. Held the interview at sister's home across the street so son would not blow up! The son was convalescing past money support point which may be a cause."

In a few of these cases there were signs that another family member, such as the husband, kept a close check on the responses to sensitive questions. These instances were important in their own right, but had only a marginal influence on the estimates of behavior patterns in the general population:

"Respondent was tired-looking. The husband remained during almost [the] entire period and paid careful attention to questions and answers. He tried to answer for the respondent at first. She was obviously very uncomfortable over the questions on violence, and I did not feel it wise to push her. I felt that the respondent was evasive on the alcohol questions; her husband corrected her several times, and she appeared to realize she was mistaken. I noticed that the respondent appeared to have a broken or missing front tooth, though she tended to keep her mouth fairly well closed, so I couldn't tell which. I had a very close feeling of violence even before the questioning began."

Objective Measures of Possible Biasing Influence of Others

There are more direct ways of studying the impact of the presence of other individuals in the interview situation, if we make certain basic assumptions about the independence of other potential explanatory variables (which we have to do in any bivariate expositions in a causal framework). The relationships between the presence of one or more "outsiders" and some central statistics of the survey are shown in Table A.6. This table does not show any clear-cut relationship between self-reported drinking behavior and the presence of other persons in the interview situation. There was definitely no tendency for respondents who were alone with the interviewer throughout the interview to report more drinking occasions or higher amounts consumed than those who were not. The same was generally true for experiences of threats and violence.

As remarked earlier, the greatest influence of a third person in an interview situation seems to be felt not on factual questions but in responses to attitude questions, questions about reasons for drinking, and so forth, where truth conditions are more vague. For some analytical purposes, this may not even be regrettable. This is so if responses to some interview items are meant to reflect decision-making and attitudinal behavior tendencies as they occur in real-life situations. Such processes do not take place in a social vacuum, as, for example, a well-known study of voting behavior found some years ago (Katz & Lazarsfeld, 1955). Here we are up against the atomistic ideals of survey research, which may conflict with social reality. However, if a study is aimed at eliciting samples of real-life events in decision making and attitude formation, this should be done systematically and in an assuredly unbiased way. This was not the case in the present study.

By way of summary, it can be stated that the presence of other people in the interview situation was surprisingly high in the present study; however, indications from other studies are that this is a more common feature of interview situations in respondents' homes than is generally reported or recognized. In this study, others were most commonly present when the respondents had difficulties with the language of the interview. However, this presence did not seem to primarily affect the responses to the questions on experiences of violence and drinking behavior of the respondent. In part this may have been due to the fact that a large proportion of the individuals present were children; no doubt also it was due in part to the fact that flash cards and coded responses were used. Analyses not presented here have shown that even in the instances where the

TABLE A.6. Self-Reported Drinking Characteristics and Experiences of Aggression during the Last 12 Months, in Relation to Presence of Other Persons in the Interview Situation

	Other person(s) present			
	At no time ($n = 521$)	Part of the time ($n = 228$)	All of the time ($n = 162$)	Total ($n = 911$)
Drank alcohol at least once a year	91.2%	96.1%	88.9%	92.0%
Drank alcohol at least once a day	5.2%	8.3%	14.2%	7.6%
Drank alcohol during past 30 days	79.7%	80.3%	79.4%	80.1%
Victimized by violence in last 12 months	9.3%	8.8%	8.0%	9.0%
Threatened with weapon or object in last 12 months	2.1%	4.4%	2.5%	2.7%
Threatened verbally with violence in last 12 months	6.5%	7.0%	6.8%	6.7%
Mean number of centiliters of 100% alcohol consumed on:	($n = 491$)	($n = 206$)	($n = 141$)	($n = 838$)[a]
Last occasion in a private home	3.6	3.6	3.2	3.5
Last occasion in a public drinking place	4.2	4.2	4.7	4.4
Occasion when most alcohol was consumed in last 30 days[b]	7.9	8.7	8.3	8.2

[a]For obvious reasons, only nonabstainers are included.
[b]For infrequent drinkers (9.1% of the nonabstainer sample), a reference period of 12 months was used.

interviewer thought that the presence of a third person affected the respondent's answers, and in cases where the interviewer detected hesitation on the part of the respondent in answering key questions, there were no discernible differences in the expected direction with regard to alcohol consumption and experiences of aggression in aggregated analyses. For lack of evidence to the contrary, the following benevolent interpretation of these findings may be appropriate: Despite what seemed like the influence of other people and hesitation in responding, the respondents generally told the truth as they saw it. There is no significant evidence to the contrary in the analyses that I have carried out.

APPENDIX B

Extracts from the Questionnaire Used in the Interview Study

1. People have suggested a number of reasons for violence in our society. I have a list of some of these here (*show Card A*). Could you give me the number printed next to the reason that you think is the most important?

Card A:
1. Poverty
2. Stresses of everyday life
3. Competition between people
4. Drugs
5. Problems in the family
6. Alcohol
7. Mental problems
8. Need for excitement
9. Lack of discipline in bringing up children

Which do you think is the second most important reason?
Which do you think is the third most important reason?

2. Now I will read you a number of statements about violence, and I would like you to tell me whether you *completely agree*, with these statements or whether you *mostly agree*, *neither agree nor disagree*, *mostly disagree*, or *completely disagree*. To make it easier (*hand respondent Card B*), you can indicate how much you agree or disagree with each statement by just giving me the number next to what best describes your feelings about the statement.

Card B:

1. Completely agree
2. Mostly agree
3. Neither agree nor disagree
4. Mostly disagree
5. Completely disagree

a. Violence in Canada has increased over the past 5 years.
b. Violence is part of some sports and should be allowed without intervention by the legal authorities.
c. Most of the people who commit murder are mentally disturbed.
d. Man is *not* aggressive by nature.
e. Alcohol is responsible for a large part of the violence in our society.
f. People who physically assault others when they are drunk should not be punished as hard as those who do so when they are sober.
g. Violence on TV is responsible for some of the violent crimes committed in Canada.
h. Some people who are not at all aggressive when they are sober can get really violent after a few drinks.
i. Children under 12 should not be allowed to watch people get killed on TV.
j. There are some areas in Thunder Bay where I do not feel safe walking around after dark.
k. There will probably be more violence in our country in the near future.
l. There is nothing wrong with slapping a child who has been disobedient.
m. Too much alcohol can make anybody violent.
n. A fist fight between two men is sometimes necessary.
o. Under no circumstances does a man have the right to beat his wife.
p. It is normal for a man to hit somebody who provokes him.
q. When a person does you wrong you should try to forgive him or her.
r. Disagreement between people can always be resolved by talking things over.

3. Now I have some questions about your personal experiences of violence. We don't want to include physical contact that is part of some sports and games or that was not intended to hurt you. Here is a list of some violent or aggressive things that can happen to people (*hand respondent Card C*). Can you tell me which of these things have happened to *you* since you were 15 years old? Include everything, whether it was done by a person you know or a stranger. Just tell me "yes" or "no" as I read the letters beside the items.

Card C:

a. Somebody hit you with some kind of object.
b. Somebody punched you (with his/her fist).

c. Somebody kicked you.
d. Somebody hurt you by throwing something at you.
e. Somebody slapped you (with his/her hand).
f. Somebody hurt you by grabbing, pushing, or shoving.
g. Somebody hurt you in some other way. Please describe!

(*If "no" to all of the above, go to question 27*)

4. Thinking back over the last 12 months, on how many different occasions has anybody hurt you physically in any of the ways listed on the card (*Card C*) or in any other way?
5. When was the last time any of these things happened to you? (*month and year*)
6. At that time, which of the things listed on the card (*Card C*) did the person (or persons) do to hurt you? Just tell me "yes" or "no" as I read the letters.
7. Where did this happen? (*Show Card D*) Please give me the number next to the kind of place.

Card D:
1. At your own home
2. In somebody else's home
3. At work or school
4. In a tavern, restaurant, or other place where alcohol is served
5. In the street or a park
6. Some other place

(*If "4" [public drinking place], ask*:) Would you mind telling me the name of this place?
(*If "6" [other], ask*:) Please describe this place.

8. Was this in the city of Thunder Bay?
(*If "no," ask*:) Where was it?
9. At approximately what time of the day or night did it take place? (*hour, A.M./P.M.*)
10. What day of the week was it?
11. Could you give me a short description of how and why this incident started? And how did it end?
12. How many people saw it happen, except for you and the other person?
13. Did any of these people try to stop what was going on?
14. Did more than one person hurt you?
(*If "yes," ask*:) How many persons were there?
(*Ask respondent to think of the main assailant in answering the following questions about the person who hurt him/her*)
15. On this card a number of characteristics to describe a person are listed

(*hand respondent Card E*). Could you please tell me how old you would estimate that the person was who hurt you? Just give me the number next to the age group.

Card E—Age:
1. Under 15 years old
2. Between 15 and 19
3. Between 20 and 29
4. Between 30 and 39
5. Between 40 and 49
6. Between 50 and 59
7. Between 60 and 69
8. Over 70 years old

16. Could you now tell me, in the same way, whether the person was male or female?

Card E—Sex:
1. Male
2. Female

17. Could you also give me the number beside the phrase that describes your relationship to this person?

Card E—Relationship to person:
1. Wife/husband
2. Mother/father
3. Sister/brother
4. Girlfriend/boyfriend
5. Somebody from work or school
6. Somebody from the neighborhood
7. Other

(*If "1," "2," or "3" go to question 19*)
(*If "7"*[*other*] *ask*:) Could you describe how you knew or met this person, in a few words?

18. Could you also tell me the number next to the phrase that best describes how well you knew the person?

Card E—How well did you know the person:
1. Very well
2. Fairly well
3. A little

4. Hardly at all
5. Not at all

19. Were you injured at all? (*If "no," go to question 21*)
20. What did you do about it? Did you . . .

a. Go to a hospital, doctor, or nurse?
b. Take or apply any medication?

21. Were the police involved at any stage? (*If "no," go to question 23*)
22. Were any charges laid?
23. Had the person who hurt you been drinking alcohol before the incident? (*If "no," or "don't know," go to question 25*)
24. Would you say that this person was drunk?
25. Had you yourself had any alcohol before this incident took place? (*If "no," or "don't remember," go to question 27*)
26. Could you tell me what you had been drinking? You can give me the approximate amount in number of glasses, bottles, or total ounces, whichever way you find easiest. Did you have any of the following:

Beer
Table wine
Dessert wine
Whisky (with or without mixer?)
Rye (with or without mixer?)
Vodka (with or without mixer?)
Gin (with or without mixer?)
Rum (with or without mixer?)
Other alcoholic beverages—please describe!

27. Now I would like to ask you a few questions about another form of aggressive behavior that you may have experienced—that is, *threats* of physical violence. When you think of your past experience, please do not include threatening remarks made jokingly. Also, don't count the occasions when you actually experienced physical violence in connection with a threat. Can you please tell me which of these things have happened to you since you were 15 years old? (*hand respondent Card F*) Just tell me "yes" or "no" as I read the letters beside the items.

Card F:
a. Somebody threatened you with a gun.
b. Somebody threatened you with a knife.
c. Somebody threatened to hurt you with some other weapon or object. Please describe!

d. Somebody said he/she was going to kill you.
e. Somebody said he/she was going to beat you up.
f. Somebody said he/she was going to hurt you in some other way. Please describe!

(*If "no" to all of the above, go to question 48*)

28. Thinking back over the last 12 months, on how many occasions has somebody threatened you with some kind of weapon? That is, how many times has a, b, or c (*Card F*) happened to you? Do not count any occasions when somebody actually hurt you with a weapon or object.

29. Again, thinking back over the last 12 months, on how many occasions has somebody said something threatening to you? That is, how many times has d, e, or f (*Card F*) happened to you? Again, do not count any occasions when somebody actually hurt you physically.

* * *

55. And now I would like to ask you a question about violence that you may have witnessed, but not been involved in yourself. Again, do not include playful aggressive behavior or physical contact that is part of some sports. Thinking back over the last 12 months, have you *seen* somebody do any of the following things to another person? (*hand respondent Card H*) Just tell me "yes" or "no" as I read the letters.

Card H:
a. Hit somebody with some kind of weapon or object.
b. Punch somebody (with his/her fist).
c. Kick somebody.
d. Hurt somebody by throwing an object.
e. Slap somebody (with his/her hand).
f. Hurt somebody by grabbing, pushing, or shoving.
g. Hurt somebody in some other way. Please describe!

(*If "no" to all of the above, go to question 59*)

56. On how many *different occasions* during the last 12 months have you seen physical violence as described on the card? (*Card H*)

57. Where have you seen these things happen during the last 12 months? (*Show Card D—see question 7*) Just tell me "yes" or "no" as I read the numbers.

58. Did all these incidents take place in the city of Thunder Bay?

59. Now we need some information about your own consumption of alcohol. First of all, how often do you yourself use alcohol? Please look at this card (*hand respondent Card I*) and tell me the number next to what best describes how often you have at least one drink of beer, wine, or spirits, or any other kind of alcohol.

Card I:

1. At least once a day
2. Nearly every day
3. Several times a week (three or four)
4. Twice a week
5. Once a week
6. About twice a month
7. About once a month
8. Less often than once a month but at least once a year
9. Less often than once a year

0. Never

(*If "9" or "0," go to question 104*)

60. Now let's look at your consumption during the past 30 days. On how many of the last 30 days have you had at least one drink of alcohol?

61. On how many of the last 30 days did you have a drink of alcohol in your own home or somebody else's home?

62. When did you last have a drink of alcohol in your own home or somebody else's home, not counting today? (*day and month*)

63. What did you drink then? You can tell me the approximate amounts in number of glasses, bottles, or total ounces, whichever way you find easiest. Did you have any . . . (*See question 26 for list of beverages*)

* * *

73. On how many days of the last 30 days did you have a drink of alcohol in a public drinking place, such as a tavern, bar, or restaurant?
(*If respondent has had at least one drink of alcohol in a public drinking place during the last 30 days, go to question 75*)

74. On how many days of the last 12 months have you had a drink of alcohol in a public drinking place?

75. People go to public drinking places for different reasons. On this card some of the reasons are listed (*hand respondent Card L*). Could you tell me what reasons are important to *you*, by telling me "yes" if the reason is important and "no" if it is not important, as I read the letters?

Card L:

a. To play games (shuffleboard, pool, etc.)
b. To eat
c. To dance
d. To see friends
e. To get some excitement
f. To talk about interesting things
g. To feel close to people

h. To have a good time
i. To meet new people
j. To watch and listen to entertainment
k. To relax after a day's work
l. To let loose, to celebrate

76. Now I would like to ask you specifically about the *last time* you had a drink of alcohol in a public drinking place, not counting today. First of all, when was this? (*day and month*)

77. Would you mind telling me what the name of the place was?

78. What did you have to drink then? Again, you can give me the approximate amounts in number of glasses, bottles, or total ounces, whichever way you find easiest. Did you have any . . . (*See question 26 for list of beverages*)

* * *

92. How much would you say was the most alcohol you drank on any one occasion during the last 30 days? (*If respondent did not have a drink of alcohol during the last 30 days, ask*:) Or during the last 12 months? Again, you can give me the approximate amounts in number of glasses, bottles, or total ounces, whichever way you find easiest. Did you have any . . . (*See question 26 for list of beverages*)

93. When was that? (*day and month*)

* * *

103. Now I am going to read a list of reasons why people drink alcohol. Could you tell me what reasons are important to *you* by telling me "yes" if the reason is important and "no" if it is not important?

a. Because it tastes good.
b. Because most of the people you know drink alcohol.
c. Because it helps you forget your problems for a while.
d. Because it is easier to talk to people after a couple of drinks.
e. Because it helps you go to sleep.
f. Because it helps you relax when you are tense or restless.
g. Because you are used to it.
h. Because it perks you up when you are tired or in a bad mood.

104. Now I am going to read some statements that have been made about alcohol and the way people behave when drinking. Could you again tell me if you agree or disagree with these statements in the same way as before? (*Hand respondent Card B—see question 2*)

a. Some men drink to have an excuse for fighting.
b. The feeling of happiness brought about by alcohol is not genuine.

c. If a man hits his wife when he is drunk, it is not as bad as if he hits her while sober.
d. If people drink alcohol, they should have one or two drinks a night instead of drinking heavily on weekends.
e. Alcohol brings out good things in many people.
f. Being drunk is something to be ashamed of.
g. A person who is drunk is not responsible for his actions.
h. Drinking hard liquor makes people more aggressive than drinking beer.
i. Sober enjoyment is the only real enjoyment.
j. Under the influence of alcohol, one is allowed to do many things that are not proper when sober.
k. A man who kills somebody while he is drunk should get the same punishment as a sober man who kills somebody.
l. Some people drink to make it easier to show their feelings.
m. If two friends get mad at each other while drinking, it should not affect their relationship when they are sober.
n. We should forgive a person more easily for what he does when he is drunk.

105. Would you say that there are areas or locations in Thunder Bay where there is more violence than most other parts of the city? If so, could you name one or more such areas or locations?

* * *

109. What do you think stops most people from physically hurting another person even when they are really angry? I would like to know whether you think the reasons I am going to read are important or not for people. Just tell me "yes" or "no" as I read them.

a. Because they are afraid of getting hurt themselves.
b. Because they are concerned about what people who see them will think.
c. Because they are concerned what their family will say.
d. Because they feel violence is wrong.
e. Because they do not want to get into trouble with the law.
f. Because they are concerned about what their friends will say.

110. And now finally, I have a few questions to ask about yourself. How long have you lived in Thunder Bay? (*Write in number of years; round off to closest full year*)

111. Have you lived most of your life in . . .

1. A city or town
2. The country

112. In what country were you born?

* * *

125. And last of all, here are a few questions to check how well our sample represents the Thunder Bay population. Please look at this card and tell me which category best describes your present status. (*Hand respondent Card O*) Just give me the number next to the category.

Card O:
1. Housewife
2. Student
3. Retired/pensioned
4. Unemployed
5. Employed
6. Other—please describe!

(*If "1" or "2" go to question 128*)

126. What is (was) your occupation?
127. And what exactly do (did) you do?
128. What is the highest level of schooling that you completed? (*Hand respondent Card P*) Just give me the letter beside your highest level.

Card P:
a. Never attended school
b. Grade 1–4
c. Grade 5–8
d. Grade 9–11
e. Grade 12–13
f. Some college/university, but no degree
g. College/university degree

129. Now please look at this card (*hand respondent Card Q*) and tell me which category includes the total income for last year, before taxes, of all the members of your household. Please just tell me the letter beside the category.

Card Q:
a. Under $1,000
b. Between $1,000 and $2,999
c. Between $3,000 and $4,999
d. Between $5,000 and $6,999
e. Between $7,000 and $9,999
f. Between $10,000 and $14,999
g. Between $15,000 and $19,999

h. Between $20,000 and $29,999
i. Over $30,000

130. What year were you born?
131. What is your marital status? Are you . . .

1. Married
2. Single
3. Separated/divorced
4. Widowed
5. Other—please describe!

132. (*Write in sex or respondent: male = 1, female = 2*)

* * *

Thank you very much.

References

Abel, E. L., & Zeidenberg, P. (1985). Age, alcohol and violent death: A postmortem study. *Journal of Studies on Alcohol, 46*, 228–231.

Aftonbladet [Stockholm, Sweden]. (1985, February 28). [Panic in the old-age home: Man in wheelchair fired pistol].

Ahlström-Laakso, S. (1973). *European drinking habits: A review of research and some suggestions for conceptual integration of findings* (Report No. 73). Helsinki: Social Research Institute of Alcohol Studies.

Aho, T. (1967). Alkoholi ja aggressiivinen käyttäytyminen [Alcohol and aggressive behavior]. *Alkoholipolitiikka, 32*, 179–184.

Aho, T. (1976). *Alkoholi ja väkivalta* [Alcohol and Violence.] (Report No. 7, D Series). Helsinki: Oikeusministeriö [Ministry of Justice].

Amaro, H., Fried, L. E., Cabral, H., & Zuckerman, B. (1990). Violence during pregnancy and substance use. *American Journal of Public Health, 80*, 575–579.

Amir, M. (1971). *Patterns in forcible rape*. Chicago: University of Chicago Press.

Anderson, E. (1978). *A place on the corner*. Chicago: University of Chicago Press.

Aromaa, K. (1977a). *Gallup-tutkimukseen perustuvia tietoja alkoholinkäytöstä ja väkivallantekojen uhriksi joutumisesta* [English summary: *Alcohol consumption and victimization to violence: Correlations in a national sample*] (Publication No. 22). Helsinki: Research Institute of Legal Policy.

Aromaa, K. (1977b). *Kolme uhritutkimusta 1970–1976: Galluptutkimuksia väkivallan uhriksi joutumisesta* [English summary: *Three victim surveys: Gallup surveys on victimization to violence*] (Publication No. 23). Helsinki: Research Institute of Legal Policy.

Asimakopulos, A. (1965). Analysis of Canadian consumer expenditure surveys. *Canadian Journal of Economics and Political Science, 31*, 222–236.

Baum-Baicker, C. (1985). The psychological benefits of moderate alcohol consumption: A review of the literature. *Drug and Alcohol Dependence, 15*, 305–322.

Behling, D. W. (1979). Alcohol abuse as encountered in 51 instances of reported child abuse. *Clinical Pediatrics, 18*, 87–91.

Bennett, R. M., Buss, A. H., & Carpenter, J. A. (1969). Alcohol and human physical aggression. *Quarterly Journal of Studies on Alcohol, 30*, 870–876.

Berger, P. L., & Luckmann, T. (1966). *The social construction of reality*. Garden City, NY: Doubleday.

Berglund, M., & Tunving, K. (1985). Assaultive alcoholics 20 years later. *Acta Psychiatrica Scandinavica, 71*, 141–147

Bergson, H. (1911). *Laughter*. London: Macmillan.

Biderman, A. D., Johnson, L. A., McIntyre, J., & Weir, A. W. (1967). Report on a pilot study in the District of Columbia on victimization and attitudes toward law enforcement. In President's Commission on Law Enforcement and Administration of Justice (Ed.). *Field surveys 1*. Washington, DC: U.S. Government Printing Office.

Bjerke, T. (1986, December 11–13). *Aggresjon som biologisk fenomen* [*Aggression as a biological phenomenon*]. Paper presented at Nordic Research Seminar on Alcohol and Violence, Bergen, Norway.

Bödal, K. (1987). 416 menn anmeldt till Oslo politikammer for kvinnemishandling: Omfanget av alkoholmisbruk i denne gruppen [Four-hundred and sixteen men reported to the police for assaults on women: The extent of alcohol abuse in this group]. In *Alkoholbruk och dess konsekvenser: Rapport från det nordiska samhällsvetenskapliga forskarmötet 1986* [Report from the Nordic Research Meeting in the Social Sciences 1986] (Publication No. 15). Helsinki: Nordic Council for Alcohol and Drug Research.

Bowden, K. M., Wilson, D. W., & Turner, L. K. (1958). A survey of blood alcohol testing in Australia (1951–1956). *Medical Journal of Australia, 2*, 13–15.

Boyatzis, R. E. (1974). The effect of alcohol consumption on the aggressive behavior of men. *Quarterly Journal of Studies on Alcohol, 35*, 959–972.

Boyatzis, R. E. (1975). The predisposition toward alcohol-related interpersonal aggression in men. *Journal of Studies on Alcohol, 36*, 1196–1207.

Brodersen, P., Larsen, T., Bendtsen, F., Larsen, A., & Ulrichsen, H. (1985). Vold mod kvinder i samlivsforhold: I. Forekomst, skademekanisme, skadetype og behandling [English summary: Violence to women in their partnerships: I. Incidence, mechanisms of injury, types of injury and treatment]. *Ugeskrift for Laeger, 147*, 1561–1564.

Bryggman, J. (1984, December 31). [Letter to the editor: Stockholm by night!]. *Dagens Nyheter* [Stockholm, Sweden].

Burns, T. F. (1980). Getting rowdy with the boys. *Journal of Drug Issues, 1*, 273–286.

Burridge, K. O. L. (1967). Lévi-Strauss and myth. In E. Leach (Ed.), *The structural study of myth and totemism*. London: Tavistock.

Bushman, B. J., & Cooper, H. M. (1990). Effects of alcohol on human aggression: An integrative research review. *Psychological Bulletin, 107*, 341–354.

Byles, J. A. (1978). Violence, alcohol problems and other problems in disintegrating families. *Journal of Studies on Alcohol, 39*, 551–553.

Byles, J. A. (1980). Family violence in Hamilton. *Canada's Mental Health, 28*, 4–6.

Cameron, T. (1977). Alcohol and traffic. In M. Aarens, T. Cameron, J. Roizen, R. Roizen, R. Room, D. Schneberk, & D. Wingard (Eds.), *Alcohol, casualties and crime* (Report No. C-18). Berkeley: Social Research Group, University of California.

Campbell, A., & Gibbs, J. J. (Eds.). (1986). *Violent transactions: The limits of personality.* Oxford: Blackwell.

Cannell, C. F., Marquis, K. H., & Laurent, A. (1977). *A summary of studies of interviewing methodology* (Vital and Health Statistics, Series 2, No. 69). Hyattsville, MD: National Center for Health Statistics.

Carlson, B. E. (1977). Battered women and their assailants. *Social Work, 22*, 455–460.

Carsjö, K. (1977). *The relationship between alcohol consumption and violent crime: Some evidence from Canada and Scandinavia.* Unpublished manuscript, Addiction Research Foundation, Toronto.

Carsjö, K. (1985). Validiteten i självrapporterat sjukvårdsutnyttjande [The validity of self-reported health care utilization]. *Socialmedicinsk tidskrift, 62*, 310–313.

Cavan, S. (1966). *Liquor license: An ethnography of bar behavior.* Chicago: Aldine.

Central Bureau of Statistics, Sweden. (1981). *Levnadsförhållanden: Offer för vålds- och egendomsbrott 1978* [*Living conditions: Victims of crimes of violence and property crimes*]. Stockholm: Author.

Central Bureau of Statistics, Sweden. (1987). *Rättstatistisk årsbok* [*Yearbook of Judicial Statistics*]. Stockholm: Author.

Cherek, D. R., Steinberg, J. L., & Manno, B. R. (1985). Effects of alcohol on human aggressive behavior. *Journal of Studies on Alcohol, 46*, 321–328.

Cherpitel, C. J. S. (1989). Breath analysis and self-reports as measures of alcohol-related emergency room admissions. *Journal of Studies on Alcohol, 50*, 155–161.

Christie, N., Andenaes, J., & Skirbekk, S. (1965). A study of self-reported crime. In K. O. Christiansen (Ed.), *Scandinavian studies in criminology* (Vol. 1). London: Tavistock.

Cohen, J. (1960). *Chance, skill and luck: The psychology of guessing and gambling.* Harmondsworth, England: Penguin Books.

Collins, J. J., & Schlenger, W. E. (1988). Acute and chronic effects of alcohol use on violence. *Journal of Studies on Alcohol, 49*, 516–521.

Connors, G. J., & Maisto, S. A. (1979). Effects of alcohol, instructions, and consumption rate on affect and physiological sensations. *Psychopharmacology, 62*, 261–266.

Criminal Justice Commission. (1967). *Criminal homicides in Baltimore, Maryland, 1960–1964: An analysis prepared by the staff of Criminal Justice Commission, Inc.* Baltimore: Author.

Dahl, E., Wickström, E., & Bo, O. (1981). Alkohol og medikamenter hos voldsofre [Alcohol and medical drugs in victims of violence]. *Tidsskrift for den Norske Laegeforening, 101*, 329–330.

Davis, H. (1987). Workplace homicides of Texas males. *American Journal of Public Health*, *77*, 1290–1293.

Dietz, P. E., & Baker, S. P. (1987). Murder at work. *American Journal of Public Health*, *77*, 1273–1274.

Eberle, P. A. (1982). Alcohol abusers and non-users: A discriminant analysis of differences between two subgroups of batterers. *Journal of Health and Social Behavior*, *23*, 260–271.

Eco, U. (1979). *A theory of semiotics*. Bloomington: Indiana University Press.

Ekman, G., Frankenhaeuser, M., Goldberg, L., Hagdahl, R., & Myrsten, A.-L. (1964). Subjective and objective effects of alcohol as functions of dosage and time. *Psychopharmacologia*, *6*, 399–409.

Ennis, P. H. (1967). Criminal victimization in the United States: Report of a National Survey. In President's Commission on Law Enforcement and Administration of Justice (Ed.). *Field surveys 2*. Washington, DC: U.S. Government Printing Office.

Epstein, T., Cameron, T., & Room, R. (1977). Alcohol and family abuse. In M. Aarens, T. Cameron, J. Roizen, R. Roizen, R. Room, D. Schneberk, & D. Wingard (Eds.), *Alcohol, casualties and crime*. (Report No. C-18). Berkeley: Social Research Group, University of California.

Erickson, M. L., & Empey, L. T. (1963). Court records, undetected delinquency and decision making. *Journal of Criminal Law, Criminology and Police Science*, *54*, 456–469.

Evans, J. L., & Leger, G. J. (1979). Canadian victimization surveys: A discussion paper. *Canadian Journal of Criminology*, *21*, 166–183.

Expressen [Stockholm, Sweden]. (1985, June 16). [This is a car ride he will not remember].

Expressen [Stockholm, Sweden]. (1988, April 27). [When the wife got excited, so did the husband].

Falk, P., & Sulkunen, P. (1981). Kulttuuri, alkoholi ja alkoholikulttuuri [Culture, alcohol and alcohol culture]. *Alkoholipolitiikka*, *46*, 314–320.

Fekjaer, H. O. (1985). Alkohol og vold [Alcohol and violence]. In H. Laake (Ed.), *Alkohol og vold*. Oslo: Universitetsforlaget.

Ferracuti, F., & Newman, G. (1974). Assaultive offenses. In D. Glaser (Ed.), *Handbook of criminology*. Chicago: Rand McNally.

Forgas, J. P. (1979). *Social episodes*. London: Academic Press.

Foster, J. (1983, March 15). [U.K. nannies get boot from pubs. Shouting and pranks highlight young ladies' nights on town]. *Toronto Star*.

Freed, E. X. (1978). Alcohol and mood: An updated review. *International Journal of the Addictions*, *13*, 173–200.

Gadourek, I. (1963). *Riskante Gewoonten en Zorg voor eigen Welzijn* [*High-risk habits and the care of one's welfare*]. Groningen, The Netherlands: Wolters.

Geertz, C. (1973). *The interpretation of cultures*. New York: Basic Books.

Gelles, R. J. (1987). *Family violence*. Beverly Hills, CA: Sage.

Germain, S., Mattila, K., Meyer-Törnroth, C., & Polkunen-Gartz, M.-L. (1980). *Våld i hemmet: en rapport om kvinnomisshandel* [*Violence in the home: A report on battering of women*]. Lovisa, Finland: Schildts.

Gerson, L. W. (1978). Alcohol-related acts of violence: Who was drinking and where the acts occurred. *Journal of Studies on Alcohol, 39*, 1204–1206.

Gerson, L. W., & Preston, D. A. (1979). Alcohol consumption and the incidence of violent crime. *Journal of Studies on Alcohol, 40*, 307–312.

Gibson, L., Linden, R., & Johnson, S. (1980). A situational theory of rape. *Canadian Journal of Criminology, 22*, 51–65.

Giesbrecht, N., Gonzalez, R., Grant, M., Osterberg, E., Room, R., Rootman, I., & Toule, L. (Eds.). (1989). *Drinking and casualties: Accidents, poisonings and violence in an international perspective.* London: Tavistock/Routledge.

Goffman, E. (1959). *The presentation of self in everyday life.* Garden City, NY: Doubleday/Anchor.

Goffman, E. (1961). *Encounters: Two studies in the sociology of interaction.* Indianapolis: Bobbs-Merrill.

Goffman, E. (1963). *Behavior in public places: Notes on the social organization of gatherings.* Glencoe, IL: Free Press.

Goffman, E. (1967). *Interaction ritual: Essays on face-to-face behavior.* Garden City, NY: Doubleday/Anchor.

Goffman, E. (1971). *Relations in public: Microstudies of the public order.* New York: Basic Books.

Goffman, E. (1974). *Frame analysis: An essay on the organization of experience.* New York: Harper & Row.

Goodman, R. A., Mercy, J. A., Loya, F., Rosenberg, M. L., Smith, J. C., Allen, N. H., Vargas, L., & Kolts, R. (1986). Alcohol use and interpersonal violence: Alcohol detected in homicide victims. *American Journal of Public Health, 76*, 144–149.

Gustafson, R. (1986a). *Alcohol and human physical aggression: The mediating role of frustration.* Uppsala, Sweden: University of Uppsala.

Gustafson, R. (1986b). Alcohol, frustration, and aggression: An experiment using the balanced placebo design. *Psychological Reports, 59*, 207–218.

Haberman, P. W., & Baden, M. M. (1978). *Alcohol, other drugs and violent death.* New York: Oxford University Press.

Hagnell, O., Nyman, E., & Tunving, K. (1973). Dangerous alcoholics: Personality varieties in aggressive and suicidally inclined subjects. *Scandinavian Journal of Social Medicine, 3*, 125–131.

Hales, T., Seligman, P. J., Newman, S. C., & Timbrook, C. L. (1988). Occupational injuries due to violence. *Journal of Occupational Medicine, 30*, 483–487.

Hansen, H. J. P. (1977). *Drab i Danmark 1946–1970* [*Criminal homicide in Denmark 1946–1970*]. Copenhagen: Munksgaard.

Hansen, H. J. P. (1985). Criminal homicide in Greenland. *Arctic Medical Research, 40*, 61–64.

Hansen, H. J. P., & Bjarnarson, Ö. (1974). Homicide in Iceland 1946–1970. *Journal of Forensic Science, 4*, 107–117.

Hartocollis, P. (1962). Drunkenness and suggestion: An experiment with intravenous alcohol. *Quarterly Journal of Studies on Alcohol, 23*, 376–389.

Heath, D. B. (1958). Drinking patterns of the Bolivian Camba. *Quarterly Journal of Studies on Alcohol, 19*, 491–508.

Heath, D. B. (1988a). Alcohol control policies and drinking patterns: An international game of politics against science. *Journal of Substance Abuse, 1*, 109–115.

Heath, D. B. (1988b). Quasi-science and public policy: A reply to Robin Room about details and misrepresentations in science. *Journal of Substance Abuse, 1*, 121–125.

Heath, D. B. (1988c). Emerging anthropological theory and models of alcohol use and alcoholism. In C. D. Chaudron & D. A. Wilkinson (Eds.), *Theories on alcoholism*. Toronto: Addiction Research Foundation.

Hedeboe, J., Charles, A. V., Nielsen, J., Grymer, F., Möller, B. N., Möller-Madsen, B., & Jensen, S. E. T. (1985). Interpersonal violence: Patterns in a Danish community. *American Journal of Public Health, 75*, 651–653.

Hindman, M. (1977). Child abuse and neglect: The alcohol connection. *Alcohol Health and Research World, 1*, 2–8.

Hood, R., & Sparks, R. (1974). *Key issues in criminology*. New York: McGraw-Hill.

Hull, J. G. (1981). A self-awareness model of the causes and effects of alcohol consumption. *Journal of Abnormal Psychology, 90*, 586–600.

Jones, B. M. (1973). Memory impairment on the ascending and descending limbs of the blood alcohol curve. *Journal of Abnormal Psychology, 82*, 24–32.

Jones, B. M., & Vega, A. (1972). Cognitive performance measured on the ascending and descending limbs of the blood alcohol curve. *Psychopharmacologica, 23*, 99–114.

Karaharju, E. O., & Stjernvall, L. (1974). The alcohol factor in accidents. *Injury, 6*, 67–69.

Katz, E., & Lazarsfeld, P. (1955). *Personal influence*. Glencoe, IL: Free Press.

Kilty, K. M. (1982). Scientific ideologies and conceptions of drinking behavior and alcoholism. *Journal of Sociology and Social Welfare, 9*, 755–765.

Kish, L. (1965). *Survey sampling*. New York: Wiley.

Kraus, J. F. (1987). Homicide while at work: Persons, industries, and occupations at high risk. *American Journal of Public Health, 77*, 1285–1289.

Kühlhorn, E. (Ed.). (1984). *Den svenska våldsbrottsligheten* [*Violent Crimes in Sweden*] (Report No. 1984:1). Stockholm: Brottsförebyggande Rådet.

Kuusi, P. (1957). *Alcohol sales experiment in rural Finland*. Helsinki: Finnish Foundation for Alcohol Studies.

Lang, A., Goeckner, D., Adesso, V., & Marlatt, A. (1975). Effects of alcohol on aggression in male social drinkers. *Journal of Abnormal Psychology, 84*, 508–518.

Langer, S. (1951). *Philosophy in a new key*. Cambridge, MA: Harvard University Press.

Lemmens, P., Knibbe, R. A., & Tan, F. (1988). Weekly recall and diary estimates of alcohol consumption in a general population survey. *Journal of Studies on Alcohol, 49*, 131–135.

Lenke, L. (1982, Fall). Alcohol and crimes of violence: A causal analysis. *Contemporary Drug Problems*, pp. 355–365.

Lenke, L. (1989). *Alcohol and criminal violence: Time series analyses in a comparative perspective*. Stockholm: Akademitryck.

Leppä, S. (1974). *A review of robberies in Helsinki in 1963–1973* (Publication No. 2). Helsinki: Research Institute of Legal Policy.

Le Roux, L. C., & Smith, I. S. (1964). Violent deaths and alcoholic intoxication. *Journal of Forensic Medicine, 11*, 131–147.

Lindström, J. (1988, May 19). [Drama on a SAS flight: "We expected the liquor to burst into flames"]. *Expressen* [Stockholm, Sweden].

Liss, G. M., & Craig, C. A. (1990). Homicide in the workplace in Ontario: Occupations at risk and limitations of existing data sources. *Canadian Journal of Public Health, 81*, 10–15.

Löberg, T. (1983). Belligerence in alcohol dependence. *Scandinavian Journal of Psychology, 24*, 285–292.

Loftus, E. F., & Marburger, W. (1983). Since the eruption of Mt. St. Helens has anyone beaten you up? Improving the accuracy of retrospective reports with landmark events. *Memory & Cognition, 11*, 114–120.

Lorenz, K. (1966). *On aggression*. London: Methuen.

MacAndrew, C., & Edgerton, R. B. (1969). *Drunken comportment*. Chicago: Aldine.

Macdonald, J. M. (1967). Homicidal threats. *American Journal of Psychiatry, 124*, 475–482.

Macrory, B. E. (1952). The tavern and the community. *Quarterly Journal of Studies on Alcohol, 13*, 609–637.

Mäkelä, K. (1971). *Measuring the consumption of alcohol in the 1968–1969 alcohol consumption study*. Helsinki: Social Research Institute of Alcohol Studies.

Malterud, K. (1982). Mishandlede kvinners skadesmönster og livssituation. *Tidsskrift for den Norske Laegeforening, 33*, 1787–1790.

Marek, Z., Widacki, J., & Hanausek, T. (1974). Alcohol as a victimogenic factor in robberies. *Forensic Science, 4*, 119–123.

Marquis, K. H., Marquis, M. S., & Polich, J. M. (1986). Response bias and reliability in sensitive topic research. *Journal of the American Statistical Association, 81*, 381–389.

McClintock, F. H. (1963). *Crimes of violence*. London: Macmillan.

McClintock, F. H. (1975). *Demographic aspects of violence*. Paper presented at a Workshop on Violence in Canadian Society, Centre of Criminology, University of Toronto.

McCollam, J. B., Burish, T. G., Maisto, S. A., & Sobell, M. B. (1980). Alcohol's effects on physiological arousal and self-reported affect and sensations. *Journal of Abnormal Psychology, 89*, 224–233.

McGuire, W. J. (1973). The yin and the yang of progress in social psychology: Seven koan. *Journal of Personality and Social Psychology, 26*, 446–456.

Meyerson, A. (1959). Alcoholism: The role of social ambivalence. In R. McCarthy (Ed.), *Drinking and intoxication*. New York: Free Press.

Midanik, L. (1982). The validity of self-reported alcohol consumption and alcohol problems: A literature review. *British Journal of Addiction, 77*, 357–382.
Miller, B. A., Downs, W. R., & Gondoli, D. M. (1989). Spousal violence among alcoholic women as compared to a random household sample of women. *Journal of Studies on Alcohol, 50*, 533–540.
Ministry of Supply and Services Canada. (1982). *1981 census of Canada.* (Statistics Canada, Government Publication No. E-485). Ottawa: Author.
Ministry of Supply and Services Canada. (1983). *1981 census of Canada. Census division and subdivisions: Selected social and economic characteristics, Ontario.* Ottawa: Author.
Ministry of Supply and Services Canada. (1984a). *1981 census of Canada. Population: Language, ethnic origin, religion, place of birth, schooling* (Catalogue No. 93-950, Vol. 2). Ottawa: Author.
Ministry of Supply and Services Canada. (1984b). *1981 census of Canada. Population* (Catalogue No. 93-966, Vol. 2). Ottawa: Author.
Möller-Madsen, B., Dalgaard, J. B., Charles, A. V., Grymer, F., Hedeboe, J., Jensen, S. E. T., Möller, B. N., Nielsen, J., & Sommer, J. (1986). Alcohol involvement in violence: A study from a Danish community. *Zeitschrift für Rechtsmedizin, 97*, 141–146.
Morgan, M. M., & Steedman, D. J. (1986). Violence and the accident and emergency department. *Health Bulletin, 43*, 278–282.
Murdoch, D., & Pihl, R. O. (1985). Alcohol and aggression in group interaction. *Addictive Behaviors, 10*, 97–101.
Myrsten, A.-L. (1971). *Effects of alcohol on psychological functions* (Supplement No. 7). Stockholm: Psychological Laboratories, University of Stockholm.
Nisbett, R. (1976). *Sociology as an art form.* New York: Oxford University Press.
Normandeau, A. (1968). *Trends and patterns in crimes of robbery.* Ann Arbor, MI: University Microfilms International.
Nowlis, V. (1965). Research with the Mood Adjective Check List. In S. S. Tomkins & C. Izard (Eds.), *Affect, cognition and personality.* New York: Springer.
Olsson, O., & Wikström, P.-O. H. (1982, Fall). Effects of the experimental Saturday closing of liquor retail stores in Sweden. *Contemporary Drug Problems*, pp. 325–353.
Partanen, J. (1980). *Finnish intoxication on the screen* (Report No. 143). Helsinki: Social Research Institute of Alcohol Studies.
Paul, D. M. (1975). Drugs and aggression. *Medicine, Science and Law, 15*, 16–21.
Pernanen, K. (1974). Validity of survey data on alcohol use. In R. J. Gibbins, Y. Israel, H. Kalant, R. E. Popham, W. Schmidt, & R. G. Smart (Eds.), *Research advances in alcohol and drug problems.* New York: Wiley.
Pernanen, K. (1976). Alcohol and crimes of violence. In B. Kissin & H. Begleiter (Eds.), *The biology of alcoholism: Vol. 4. Social aspects of alcoholism.* New York: Plenum Press.
Pernanen, K. (1981). Theoretical aspects of the relationship between alcohol and crime. In J. J. Collins (Ed.), *Drinking and crime.* New York: Guilford Press.

Pernanen, K. (1985). *Survey reporting on experiences of aggression*. Unpublished manuscript.

Pernanen, K. (1989a). Remarks on causal inferences and the role of alcohol in accidents, poisonings and violence. In N. Giesbrecht, R. Gonzalez, M. Grant, E. Osterberg, R. Room, I. Rootman, & L. Toule (Eds.), *Drinking and casualties: Accidents, poisonings and violence in an international perspective*. London: Tavistock/Routledge.

Pernanen, K. (1989b). *Determinants of alcohol involvement in aggression*. Unpublished manuscript.

Pernanen, K., & Carsjö, K. (1981). *Alcohol and aggressive behaviour: Report on a community study*. (Report submitted to Health and Promotion Directorate, Health and Welfare Canada). Toronto: Addiction Research Foundation.

Pihl, R. O., Smith, M., & Farrell, B. (1984). Alcohol and aggression in men: A comparison of brewed and distilled beverages. *Journal of Studies on Alcohol, 45*, 278–282.

Pittman, D. J., & Handy, W. (1964). Patterns in criminal aggravated assault. *Journal of Criminal Law, Criminology and Police Science, 55*, 462–470.

Pittman, D. J. (1967). International overview: Social and cultural factors in drinking patterns, pathological and nonpathological. In D. J. Pittman (Ed.), *Alcoholism*. New York: Harper & Row.

Pliner, P., & Cappell, H. (1974). Modification of affective consequences of alcohol: A comparison of social and solitary drinking. *Journal of Abnormal Psychology, 83*, 418–425.

Poikolainen, K., & Kärkkäinen, P. (1983). Diary gives more accurate information about alcohol consumption than questionnaire. *Drug and Alcohol Dependence, 11*, 209–216.

Powers, R. J. (1986). Aggression and violence in the family. In A. Campbell & J. J. Gibbs (Eds.), *Violent transactions: The limits of personality*. Oxford: Blackwell.

President's Commission on Crime in the District of Columbia. (1966). *Report of the President's Commission on Crime in the District of Columbia*. Washington, DC: U.S. Government Printing Office.

Prus, R. C. (1978). From barrooms to bedrooms: Towards a theory of interpersonal violence. In M. A. B. Gammon (Ed.), *Violence in Canada*. Toronto: Methuen.

Raivio, Y. (1975). *Kanadan Suomalaisten historia* [*The history of Finns in Canada*]. Vancouver: New West Press.

Reiss, A. J., Jr. (1967). Studies in crime and law enforcement in major metropolitan areas. In President's Commission on Law Enforcement and Administration of Justice (Ed.). *Field surveys 3* (Vol. 1). Washington, DC: U.S. Government Printing Office.

Renson, G. J., Adams, J. E., & Tinklenberg, J. R. (1978). Buss-Durkee assessment and validation with violent versus nonviolent chronic alcohol abusers. *Journal of Consulting and Clinical Psychology, 46*, 360–361.

Richardson, D. C. (1980). Alcohol and wife abuse: The effect of alcohol on attributions of blame for wife abuse. *Personality and Social Psychology Bulletin*, *6*, 51–56.

Roebuck, J. B., & Frese, W. (1976). *The Rendez-Vous: A case study of an after-hours club*. New York: Free Press.

Roizen, J., & Schneberk, D. (1977). Alcohol and crime. In M. Aarens, T. Cameron, J. Roizen, R. Roizen, R. Room, D. Schneberk, & D. Wingard (Eds.), *Alcohol, casualties and crime* (Report No. C-18). Berkeley: Social Research Group, University of California.

Room, R. (1976). Ambivalence as a sociological explanation: The case of cultural explanations of alcohol problems. *American Sociological Review*, *41*, 1047–1065.

Room, R. (1987). Relating drinking and drugs to injury control: Perspectives and prospects. *Public Health Reports*, *102*, 617–620.

Room, R. (1988). Science is in the details: Towards a nuanced view of alcohol control studies. *Journal of Substance Abuse*, *1*, 117–120.

Roslund, B., & Larson, C. A. (1979). Crimes of violence and alcohol abuse in Sweden. *International Journal of the Addictions*, *14*, 1103–1115.

Roy, M. (1977). Current survey of 150 cases. In M. Roy (Ed.), *Battered women*. New York: Van Nostrand Reinhold.

Russell, J. A., & Mehrabian, A. (1975). The mediating role of emotions in alcohol use. *Journal of Studies on Alcohol*, *36*, 1508–1536.

Sariola, S. (1956). *Drinking patterns in Finnish Lapland*. Helsinki: Finnish Foundation for Alcohol Studies.

SAS Institute Inc. (1985). *SAS® User's Guide: Statistics, Version 5 Edition*. Cary, NC: SAS Institute Inc.

Schlesselman, J. J. (1982). *Case-control studies: Design, conduct, analysis*. New York: Oxford University Press.

Schmutte, G. T., & Taylor, S. P. (1980). Physical aggression as a function of alcohol and pain feedback. *Journal of Social Psychology*, *110*, 235–244.

Schött, S. (1988, January 22). [Clergyman exposed himself]. *Aftonbladet* [Stockholm, Sweden].

Schuckit, M. A., & Russell, J. W. (1984). An evaluation of primary alcoholics with histories of violence. *Journal of Clinical Psychiatry*, *45*, 3–6.

Schumacher, D. (1923). Alcohol as a cause of accidents. *Journal of the American Medical Association*, *8*, 2128–2129.

Senay, E. C., & Wettstein, R. (1983). Drugs and homicide: A theory. *Drug and Alcohol Dependence*, *12*, 157–166.

Simpura, J. (1983). *Drinking contexts and social meanings of drinking: A study with Finnish drinking occasions* (Vol. 33). Helsinki: Finnish Foundation for Alcohol Studies.

Skog, O.-J. (1986). Trends in alcohol consumption and violent deaths. *British Journal of Addiction*, *81*, 365–379.

Skog, O.-J. (1987, September 14–18). *Testing causal hypotheses about correlated trends: Pitfalls and remedies*. Paper presented at the Research Conference on Statistical Recording Systems of Alcohol Problems, Helsinki.

Skogan, W. G. (1977). Dimensions of the dark figure of unreported crime. *Crime and Delinquency*, *23*, 41–50.

Smith, R. C., Parker, E. S., & Noble, E. P. (1975). Alcohol and affect in dyadic social interaction. *Psychosomatic Medicine*, *37*, 25–40.

Smith, S. M., Goodman, R. A., Thacker, S. B., Burton, A. H., Parsons, J. E., & Hudson, P. (1989). Alcohol and fatal injuries: Temporal patterns. *American Journal of Preventive Medicine*, *5*, 296–302.

Söderlund, A. (1984, April 6). [Famous smile provoked holiday celebrators]. *Dagens Nyheter* [Stockholm, Sweden].

Solicitor General, Canada. (1983). *Canadian Urban Victimization Survey, Bulletin 1: Victims of crime*. Ottawa: Author.

Solicitor General, Canada. (1984). *Canadian Urban Victimization Survey, Bulletin 2: Reported and unreported crimes*. Ottawa: Author.

Solicitor General, Canada. (1985a). *Canadian Urban Victimization Survey, Bulletin 4: Female victims of crime*. Ottawa: Author.

Solicitor General, Canada. (1985b). *Canadian Urban Victimization Survey, Bulletin 6: Criminal victimization of elderly Canadians*. Ottawa: Author.

Somander, L. (1979). *Dödsfall till följd av våldsbrott i Sverige 1976, kvinnor i brottssituationen* [*Fatalities due to crimes of violence in Sweden in 1976: Women in the crime situation*]. Linköping: University of Linköping.

Spiller, N. (1982, December 12). [Sid Caesar isn't a monster anymore]. *Toronto Star*.

Statistics Canada. (1976). *Homicide in Canada: A statistical synopsis*. Ottawa: Author.

Statistics Canada. (1978a). *Census tracts, population and housing characteristics: Thunder Bay*. Ottawa: Author.

Statistics Canada. (1978b). *Crime and traffic enforcement statistics 1976*. Ottawa: Author.

Statistics Canada. (1979). *Crime and traffic enforcement statistics 1977*. Ottawa: Author.

Statistics Canada. (1980). *Crime and traffic enforcement statistics 1978*. Ottawa: Author.

Statistics Canada. (1981). *Crime and traffic enforcement statistics 1979*. Ottawa: Author.

Statistics Canada. (1982). *Crime and traffic enforcement statistics 1980*. Ottawa: Author.

Statistics Canada. (1983). *Crime and traffic enforcement statistics 1981*. Ottawa: Author.

Statistics Canada. (1984). *Crime and traffic enforcement statistics 1982*. Ottawa: Author.

Statistics Canada. (1985). *Crime and traffic enforcement statistics 1983*. Ottawa: Author.

Statistics Canada. (1986). *Crime and traffic enforcement statistics 1984*. Ottawa: Author.

Statistics Canada. (1987). *Crime and traffic enforcement statistics 1985*. Ottawa: Author.

Steele, C. M., & Southwick, L. (1985). Alcohol and social behavior: I. The psychology of drunken excess. *Journal of Personality and Social Psychology*, *48*, 18–34.

Straus, M. A. (1986a, June). Domestic violence and homicide antecedents. *Bulletin of the New York Academy of Medicine*, *62*, 446–465.

Straus, M. A. (1986b, June). Medical care costs of intrafamily assault and homicide. *Bulletin of the New York Academy of Medicine*, *62*, 556–561.

Straus, M. A., Gelles, R. J., & Steinmetz, M. (1980). *Behind closed doors: Violence in the American family*. Garden City, NY: Doubleday/Anchor.

Takala, H. (1973). Alkoholstrejkens inverkan på uppdagad brottslighet [The effect of the alcohol strike on detected crime]. *Alkoholpolitik*, *36*, 14–16.

Tardif, G. (1966). *La criminalité de violence*. Unpublished master's thesis, University of Montreal.

Tardif, G. (1967). *Les délits de violence à Montréal*. Paper presented at the Fifth Research Conference on Criminality and Deliquency, Quebec Society of Criminality, Quebec.

Taylor, S. P., Gammon, C. B., & Capasso, D. R. (1976). Aggression as a function of the interaction of alcohol and threat. *Journal of Personality and Social Psychology*, *34*, 938–41..

Taylor, S. P., & Leonard, K. E. (1983). Alcohol and human physical aggression. In R. G. Geen & E. I. Donnerstein (Eds.), *Aggression: Theoretical and empirical reviews. Vol. 2. Issues in research*. New York: Academic Press.

Taylor, S. P., Schmutte, G. T., & Leonard, K. E. (1977). Physical aggression as a function of alcohol and frustration. *Bulletin of the Psychonomic Society*, *9*, 217–218.

Taylor, W. B. (1979). *Drinking, homicide and rebellion in colonial Mexican villages*. Stanford, CA: Stanford University Press.

Toronto Star. (1978, August 30). [Mob from village attacks motorbikers with guns, clubs].

Toronto Star. (1979, January 26). [Raped woman at gunpoint: man's prison term doubled].

Toronto Star. (1979, November 17). [Ex-leader fired shots].

Toronto Star. (1980, February 2). [Man gets 1 year in pal's slaying].

Toronto Star. (1980, June 9). [Drunk guard tries to attack president].

Toronto Star. (1981, October 8). [Home brew blamed for $200,000 rampage].

Toronto Star. (1981, October 13). [Oliver Reed on assault charge after bar brawl].

Toronto Star. (1983, May 4). [Drug-crazed driver was one-man wrecking crew].

Toronto Star. (1985, April 17). [Woman in bar fight with former champ had "great left hook"].

Toronto Star. (1985, September 12). [17 policemen called to quell Cobourg chair-tossing brawl].

Toronto Star. (1987, October 16). [Drinker jailed after tour boat taken for ride].

U.S. Department of Justice, Law Enforcement Assistance Administration, National Criminal Justice Information and Statistics Service. (1977). *Criminal victimization surveys in Miami: A national crime survey report*. Washington, DC: U.S. Government Printing Office.

U.S. Department of Justice, Law Enforcement Assistance Administration, National Criminal Justice Information and Statistics Service. (1975, July). *Census of state correctional facilities: 1974 advance report*. Washington, DC: U.S. Government Printing Office.

Van Hasselt, V. B., Morrison, R. L., & Bellack, A. S. (1985). Alcohol use in wife abusers and their spouses. *Addictive Behaviors, 10*, 127–135.

Verhaege, A., & Schodet, R. (1959). Consideration sur le dosages d'alcoolemie par prelevement systematique chez les blessés. *Lille Médicale, 4*, 866.

Verkko, V. (1951). *Homicides and suicides in Finland and their dependence on the national character*. Copenhagen: G.E.C. Gads Forlag.

Virkkunen, M. (1974). Alcohol as a factor precipitating aggression and conflict behavior leading to homicide. *British Journal of Addiction, 69*, 149–154.

Vuchinich, R. E., Tucker, J. A., & Sobell, M. A. (1979). Alcohol, expectancy, cognitive labeling, and mirth. *Journal of Abnormal Psychology, 88*, 641–651.

Warr, P. (1977). Aided experiments in social psychology. *Bulletin of the British Psychological Society, 30*, 2–8.

Washburne, C. (1961). *Primitive drinking*. New York: College and University Press.

Wasikhongo, J. (1976). Uniformities in aggravated assaults in St. Louis, Mo. and Mombasa, Kenya. *International Journal of Criminology and Penology, 4*, 9–24.

Welte, J. W., & Abel, E. L. (1989). Homicide: Drinking by the victim. *Journal of Studies on Alcohol, 50*, 197–201.

Wentworth, H., & Flexner, S. B. (1974). *The pocket dictionary of American slang*. New York: Simon & Schuster.

Westermeyer, J., & Brantner, J. (1972). Violent death and alcohol use. *Minnesota Medicine, 55*, 749–752.

Wikström, P.-O. (1980). *Våldsbrott i Gävle* [*Violent crime in Gävle*]. Stockholm: Institute of Criminology, University of Stockholm.

Wikström, P.-O. (1985). *Everyday violence in contemporary Sweden: Situational and ecological aspects*. Stockholm: National Council for Crime Prevention.

Wilson, P. (1981). Improving the methodology of drinking surveys. *The Statistician, 30*, 159–167.

Winch, P. (1958). *The ideal of a social science and its relation to philosophy*. London: Routledge & Kegan Paul.

Wingard, D., & Room, R. (1977). Alcohol and home, industrial and recreational accidents. In M. Aarens, T. Cameron, J. Roizen, R. Roizen, R. Room, D. Schneberk, & D. Wingard (Eds.), *Alcohol, casualties and crime* (Report No. C-18). Berkeley: Social Research Group, University of California.

Wolfgang, M. E. (1958). *Patterns in criminal homicide*. New York: Wiley.

Wolfgang, M. E., & Singer, S. I. (1978). Victim categories of crime. *Journal of Criminal Law and Criminology, 69*, 379–394.

Yankofsky, G., Wilson, T. G., Adler, J. L., Hay, W. M., & Vrana, S. (1986). The effect of alcohol on self-evaluation and perception of negative interpersonal feedback. *Journal of Studies on Alcohol, 47*, 26–33.

Zacker, J., & Bard, M. (1977). Further findings on assaultiveness and alcohol use in interpersonal disputes. *American Journal of Community Psychology*, *5*, 373–383.

Zeichner, A., & Pihl, R. O. (1979). Effects of alcohol and behavior contingencies on human aggression. *Journal of Experimental Research in Personality*, *88*, 153–160.

Zeichner, A., & Pihl, R. O. (1980). Effects of alcohol and instigator intent on human aggression. *Journal of Studies on Alcohol*, *41*, 265–276.

Zuber, T. G. (1974). *Introduction to Canadian Criminal Law*. Toronto: McGraw-Hill Ryerson.

Index